Partnerships for Public Health and Well-being

Interagency Working in Health and Social Care
Edited by Jon Glasby

Aimed at students and practitioners, this series provides an introduction to inter-agency working across the health and social care spectrum, bringing together an appreciation of the policy background with a focus on contemporary themes. The books span a wide range of health and social care services and the impact that these have on people's lives, as well as offering insightful accounts of the issues facing professionals in a fast-changing organizational landscape.

Exploring how services and sectors interact and could change further, and the evidence for 'what works', the series is designed to frame debate as well as promote positive ways of interdisciplinary working.

Published titles

French/Swain: *Working with Disabled People in Policy and Practice*
Kellett: *Children's Perspectives on Integrated Services: Every Child Matters in Policy and Practice*
Williams: *Learning Disability Policy and Practice: Changing Lives?*
Baggott: *Partnerships for Public Health and Wellbeing: Policy and Practice*

Partnerships for Public Health and Well-being
Policy and Practice

Rob Baggott

palgrave
macmillan

First published 2013 by
PALGRAVE MACMILLAN

Palgrave Macmillan in the UK is an imprint of Macmillan Publishers Limited, registered in England, company number 785998, of Houndmills, Basingstoke, Hampshire RG21 6XS.

Palgrave Macmillan in the US is a division of St Martin's Press LLC, 175 Fifth Avenue, New York, NY 10010.

Palgrave Macmillan is the global academic imprint of the above companies and has companies and representatives throughout the world.

Palgrave® and Macmillan® are registered trademarks in the United States, the United Kingdom, Europe and other countries.

ISBN: 978–0–230–20225–2 paperback

This book is printed on paper suitable for recycling and made from fully managed and sustained forest sources. Logging, pulping and manufacturing processes are expected to conform to the environmental regulations of the country of origin.

A catalogue record for this book is available from the British Library.

A catalog record for this book is available from the Library of Congress.

Typeset by Aardvark Editorial Limited, Metfield, Suffolk
Printed and bound by TJ International Ltd, Padstow, Cornwall

Contents

List of boxes and figures

Boxes

Figures

Acknowledgements

I would like to thank the following people who have helped in various ways with this book: Series editor, Professor Jon Glasby (Director of the Health Services Management Centre, Birmingham University); Palgrave editor, Catherine Gray and editorial assistant, India Annette-Woodgate; Carrie Walker, Julie Lankester, Linda Norris and the team at Aardvark Editorial; Dr Chris Nottingham (Glasgow Caledonian University); and two of my De Montfort colleagues, Dr Kathryn Jones (for commenting on an earlier draft) and Suzanne Walker (for compiling the abbreviations). Thanks also go to Dr Michaela Willmott for allowing me to draw on findings from her excellent PhD thesis. Finally, I would like to express my thanks to Deb, Mark, Dan and Mel, and 'AJ' – Auntie Joan Clark – for their constant support and encouragement.

ROB BAGGOTT,
Leicester, March 2013

The author and publisher would like to thank Duke University Press, Suzanne Ross and Cathy Charles for their permission to use 'Dimensions of lay participation in health care decision making' (Charles and De Maio, 1993, Figure 1: Dimensions of lay participation in healthcare decision making, p. 891 in *Journal of Health Politics, Policy and Law*, 18(4)).

List of abbreviations

ACHCEW	Association of Community Health Councils for England and Wales
BINGO	Business interest non-government organization
BSE	Bovine spongiform encephalopathy
C4L	Change4Life
CAA	Comprehensive Area Assessment
CCG	Clinical Commissioning Group
CDCP	Centres for Disease Control and Prevention
CHC	Community Health Council
CHP	Community Health Partnership
COREPER	Committee of Permanent Representatives
CPP	Community Planning Partnership
CPPIH	Commission for Patient and Public Involvement in Health
CQC	Care Quality Commission
CSR	Corporate social responsibility
DH	Department of Health
DPH	Director of Public Health
EU	European Union
FSA	Food Standards Agency
GAVI	Global Alliance for Vaccines and Immunisation
GOR	Government Office for the Region
GP	General practitioner
HAZ	Health Action Zone
HCPO	Health consumer and patients' organization
HIV/AIDS	Human immunodeficiency virus/acquired immune deficiency syndrome
HLC	Healthy Living Centre
HOSC	Health Overview and Scrutiny Committee
HOTN	*(The) Health of the Nation*
ICAS	Independent Complaints Advocacy Service
IMF	International Monetary Fund
JHWS	Joint Health and Wellbeing Strategy
JSNA	Joint Strategic Needs Assessment
LA21	Local Agenda 21
LAA	Local Area Agreement
LETB	Local Education and Training Board
LGA	Local Government Association

LHRP	Local Health Resilience Partnership
LINk	Local Involvement Network
LSP	Local Strategic Partnership
NAO	National Audit Office
NAVCA	National Association for Voluntary and Community Action
NCD	Non-communicable disease
NGO	Non-government organization
NICE	National Institute for Health and Care Excellence (formerly National Institute for Health and Clinical Excellence)
NHS	National Health Service
OCS	Office for Civil Society
OECD	Organisation for Economic Co-operation and Development
OFSTED	Office for Standards in Education, Children's Services and Skills
OMC	Open Method of Coordination
OTS	Office of the Third Sector
PALS	Patient Advice and Liaison Service
PCT	Primary Care Trust
PINGO	Public interest non-government organization
PPIF	Patient and Public Involvement Forum
RD	Responsibility Deal
SARS	Severe acute respiratory syndrome
SHA	Strategic Health Authority
TB	Tuberculosis
UN	United Nations
UNEP	United Nations Environment Program
UNESCO	United Nations Educational Scientific and Cultural Organization
UNICEF	United Nations Children's Fund
VHS	Voluntary Health Scotland
WEF	World Economic Forum
WHO	World Health Organization
WTO	World Trade Organization

1 Partnerships for public health and well-being

Introduction

The purpose of this book is to explore partnerships in the field of public health and well-being. Its central focus is upon the establishment of partnerships, their rationale, practices, relationships, the problems they face, and how these can be understood and addressed. This chapter is in three parts. First, there is an examination of the rationale for partnerships in the context of public health and well-being. Second, an analysis of the historical context of partnership in this field is undertaken, which identifies key themes to be explored in later chapters. Third, key concepts and frameworks relating to the analysis of partnership and collaborative working are explored.

Public health and well-being

Although there is disagreement about the precise meaning of public health, there is consensus that at its heart lies a collective and collaborative enterprise. Rosen (1993, p. 1) observed that 'throughout human history, the major problems of health that men have faced have been concerned with community life'. Even in modern times, when individualism and consumerism have exerted a powerful influence over how we conceptualize and respond to social problems, public health is an area where collective action is still acknowledged as being extremely important (Cm 289, 1988; Wanless, 2004; Nuffield Council on Bioethics, 2007). In this context, collective action is much broader than the state acting on behalf of the community. Although state institutions do have an important role to play in public health, so do others, such as the voluntary sector and commercial organizations. Furthermore, individual citizens and communities have a key part to play in health improvement and protection.

The case for a broad, inclusive, collective approach to public health was rooted in the World Health Organization's (WHO) definition of health as a 'state of complete physical, mental and social wellbeing and not merely the absence of disease or infirmity' (WHO, 1946, p. 100). The emergence of a salutogenic paradigm (Antonovsky, 1979, 1996) further highlighted the importance of well-being (Felce and Perry, 1995; Kahneman et al., 2003; Huppert et al., 2005) and potentially widened public health to include more areas of individual and public welfare. This served to expand the scope for collective and collaborative action, bolstered by the emphasis placed by the WHO and others on 'healthy public policy', gearing public policies across different sectors to public health objectives (Milio, 1986). Healthy public policy (and the 'health in all policies' approach discussed further below) highlighted the importance of intersectoral working, bringing in actors across a wide range of policy areas (agriculture, trade, education and the environment, for example) to address health issues. It also provided a rationale for working with non-government sectors such as commerce, the voluntary sector and civil society.

A further impetus for collaborative action came from the growing interest in health inequalities and in 'social determinants' of health (WHO Commission on Social Determinants of Health, 2008; Strategic Review of Health Inequalities in England, 2010). There is much concern over the impact of social structures and material conditions on health and well-being. It is increasingly acknowledged that collaborative and intersectoral action in these policy areas, engaging with actors such as central government agencies, local government, business and voluntary and community organizations, could help to address the root causes of health inequalities and disadvantage. Furthermore, the challenge of climate change and the imperative to promote sustainable development has further highlighted the need for collaboration in public health. Modern ecological models of health place emphasis upon complex interactions that affect public health and seek to address problems and risks in an integrated way (Lang and Rayner, 2012). Collaboration is central to such action, and this is reflected in the importance given to, for example, partnership working in the field of environmental health and climate change (see, for example, UN, 1993, 2012a; WHO Regional Office for Europe, 2010).

Although collaboration is an essential ingredient of collective action in public health and well-being, it does not occur purely by chance. It is widely recognized that a proactive approach is essential, including the formation of partnerships to provide a foundation for cooperation and collaboration. Yet despite lip service being paid to its importance, effective partnership working is often very difficult to achieve in practice.

Partnerships in historical context

Problems of partnership working in public health are long-standing, and a brief historical review is worthwhile. The efforts of ancient civilizations in preventing illness are well known (Rosen, 1993). These included urban planning, sanitation and rules on hygiene. As these functions developed, political and logistical problems familiar to modern societies emerged, including the need for different authorities and sections of society to work together. For example, in Ancient Rome, specific public health functions included the supervision of public baths, the provision of water supplies, sanitation, street cleaning and food regulation, and efforts were made to integrate these functions within a coherent system of public health administration (Rosen, 1993; Robinson, 1994; Porter, 1999).

Closer to modern times, the Victorians expanded state activities in public health, but this occurred in a rather haphazard way (Hodgkinson, 1967; Wohl, 1984). Within central government, responsibilities for public health were allocated among different agencies, boards, departments and inspectorates, but there was no effective coordination of their activities (Sheard and Donaldson, 2006). There were calls for rationalization, including from the Royal Sanitary Commission in 1871. However, it was not until the creation the Ministry of Health in 1919 that comprehensive national responsibilities for public health were set out. Poor coordination and fragmentation were also found at local level. An array of different boards and committees dealt with the same underlying problems (Hodgkinson, 1967; MacDonagh, 1977). Crucially, public health administration was strongly influenced by the system of relief for the destitute, known as the Poor Law (Wohl, 1984). There was often poor liaison between Poor Law boards and other local bodies, to the detriment of public health. This was exacerbated by conflicts between professionals employed by different agencies (Hodgkinson, 1967).

During the first half of the twentieth century, state intervention in social welfare and public health increased without a corresponding improvement in collaborative governance. Both Poor Law boards and local authorities undertook disease prevention. Calls to integrate these services were ignored. For example, the Minority Report of the Royal Commission on the Poor Laws recommended the establishment of health committees at local level combining relief for the poor and sanitary functions with wide responsibilities for illness prevention and health service provision (Cd 4499, 1909). Yet it was not until 1929 that the Poor Law boards were abolished and their public health functions transferred to local authority health committees.

As local authorities became more active in public health from the late Victorian period onwards and into the early twentieth century, there was an increase in professional tensions between GPs, concerned about the encroachment of free or subsidized local services on their paid work, and the Medical Officers of Health who led local public health departments (Lewis, 1986). As a consequence, there was a poor coordination of public health services. In the interwar period, it was increasingly acknowledged that health services must be organized on a more rational basis, especially with regard to the integration of prevention and treatment (see the Dawson Report, Cmd 693, 1920), but this was not addressed.

The NHS

The creation of the NHS was in many respects a major public health achievement, extending access to comprehensive health services to the whole population, irrespective of ability to pay. It was also believed that a single national service would give greater scope for preventing illness and for integrating different services to meet health needs. However, the principal focus of the NHS was on diagnosis and treatment, leading to criticism that 'the NHS was in reality a sickness service rather than a genuine service for health' (Webster, 1996, p. 769).

Consequently, there was a lack of leadership and coordination of public health at a national level, especially after 1951 when the Ministry of Health's responsibilities for environmental health, housing, water and other public health-related services were transferred to other departments.

To make matters worse, divisions between different parts of the health service were institutionalized. The three main parts of the NHS – hospital services, family practitioners (GPs, dentists, pharmacists and opticians), and community and public health services – had separate administrative structures, and collaboration between them was poor. At this time, local authorities were responsible for managing community services, including district nursing, health visiting, ambulance services, maternity and child welfare clinics, the school health service and health education. During the 1960s, attempts were made to bring local authority community health professionals into closer contact with GPs. However, collaboration remained problematic, and for the most part hospitals, primary care and community/public health occupied different worlds.

In 1956, the Guillebaud Committee rejected incorporating local authority health services into the mainstream (Cmd 9663, 1956), although one of its members, Sir John Maude, argued that primary healthcare services should be unified under local government. In the late 1960s, the possibility of bringing the NHS under a reformed system of local government was raised by the Royal Commission on Local Government (Cmnd 4040, 1969a). In a minority report, one of the Commission's members went further, recommending the transfer of all health services to local authorities (Cm 4040, 1969b).

However, calls to integrate NHS services under local government were rejected. Instead, community health and public health services were transferred from local government to new health authorities in the NHS reorganization of 1974. Local government remained responsible for environmental health and social services. Local authorities were represented on the new area health authorities (whose boundaries were largely co-terminous with those of the shire county and metropolitan district local authorities that provided social services). A working party explored further key issues of collaboration between local government and the NHS. It recommended that duties to work together be imposed on both, and that joint committees be established to manage their interface. A statutory duty of cooperation was subsequently placed on health authorities and local councils.

Joint consultative committees were established with members drawn from health authorities and local authorities (and later, voluntary organizations). These primarily addressed, at the health–social care service interface in particular, services for people with mental illness, learning disabilities and physical disabilities, elderly people and children (Snape, 2004). Health promotion and public health issues were a legitimate topic for joint discussion (see Cmnd 7047, 1977, p. 73) but not a primary concern. The impact of the Joint Consultative Committees was marginal and variable across the country (DHSS, 1985), and they were mainly regarded as talking shops.

Attempts were made to strengthen collaboration in the late 1970s, with the creation of joint care planning teams, consisting of officers from health and local authorities. A joint finance scheme was also established to develop services,

particularly in relation to health and social care. Nonetheless, the problems of fragmentation remained and may have even become more entrenched (Wistow, 2012).
As a result, 'cooperation remained an elusive objective, belonging to the realm of
pious exhortation and utopian prospectuses' (Webster, 1996, p. 495). The situation
specifically with regard to public health was arguably even worse, given its low
profile in these arrangements.

The Thatcher and Major governments

Although the organization of public health before 1974 was imperfect, with poor
collaboration and insufficient attention to prevention and population health, it is
acknowledged that there had been a further deterioration by the mid-1980s
(Lewis, 1986; Webster, 1996; Hunter et al., 2010). Another NHS reorganization in
1982, undertaken by the Thatcher government, was criticized for undermining
collaboration by abolishing area health authorities (most of which, as noted, had
common boundaries with shire county and metropolitan district councils). As
with all reorganizations, there was also a potential disruptive effect on partnerships
as personnel and organizations changed, although this seems to have been short
term (DHSS, 1985). In addition, the Thatcher government was reluctant to
acknowledge public health issues that might otherwise have stimulated efforts to
promote collaboration. It chose to ignore the role of socioeconomic factors in
health and illness and refused to commit to a comprehensive public health strategy.
This stance effectively discouraged collaborative working in areas such as health
inequalities, as well as on lifestyle issues such as smoking, alcohol and diet.

Even so, health authorities were exhorted to produce health promotion and
prevention strategies and to work with local authorities and others on these issues
(DHSS, 1981). Policy documents on primary care emphasized the importance of
prevention and the need for all parts of the health service to work together to
improve health (Cm 249, 1987). Furthermore, following two major communicable disease outbreaks in the mid-1980s (Cmnd 9716, 1986; Cmnd 9772, 1986),
which revealed shortcomings in local public health arrangements including poor
collaboration, an inquiry was established to review the public health function,
headed by the Chief Medical Officer, Sir Donald Acheson (Cm 289, 1988). A key
theme of its report was that public health responsibilities at local level were
unclear. It recommended that the Secretary of State for Health should consider
issuing guidance to clarify and emphasize the public health responsibilities of
health authorities. Each district health authority should appoint a named leader
of the public health function (the Director of Public Health [DPH]) whose duties
would include coordination of the control of communicable disease and liaison
with other bodies, including local authorities, on public health matters. The
Acheson Report acknowledged that stronger collaboration between local
government and the NHS was needed. It recommended that the DPH and the
local authority's Chief Environmental Health Officer establish clear and regular
channels of communication.

In the late 1980s, the government came under further attack for its handling of
several high-profile health scares, mostly connected with food safety. These

included salmonella in eggs, listeria in cheese and pâtés, and the beginnings of concern about BSE (or 'mad cow disease'). These issues exposed a poor strategic management of public health issues within central government, including inter-departmental conflict, a poor use of scientific expertise, a willingness to concede to commercial interests and a failure to understand the strength of concern among the public and the media. Other issues, such as nutrition, alcohol abuse and smoking, exposed cross-departmental battles and the suppression of health consid-erations due to commercial lobbying (Taylor, 1984; Cannon, 1987; Baggott, 1990; Mills, 1992; Webster, 1996). Although on some issues, notably HIV/AIDS, the government was praised for an effective and well-coordinated response (Berridge, 1996), it lacked a coherent and comprehensive strategy on public health (Smith and Jacobson, 1988).

By the early 1990s, some partnership working on health was evident at local level. Local initiatives were inspired by the WHO's Healthy Cities movement and by Health for All (see Chapter 2). Another impetus was Local Agenda 21 (LA21), which emerged from the 'Earth Summit' held in Rio de Janeiro in 1992 (UN, 1993). LA21 encouraged local authorities to work with other local agencies and the community to improve the environment and promote sustainable develop-ment across a range of policy issues, including health. However, efforts to coord-inate action on public health were weakened by the absence of a national policy framework. This was addressed by the Major government, which formulated *The Health of the Nation* (HOTN) strategy for England (Cm 1986, 1992). This outlined a range of health targets covering the major causes of ill health and death (coro-nary heart disease and stroke, cancer, mental health, HIV/AIDs and sexual health, and accidents) alongside risk factor targets related to health behaviours and condi-tions (such as diet and nutrition, smoking, HIV/AIDs and blood pressure).

HOTN outlined how different organizations could contribute to improve-ments in health. A clear role for central government was identified, with an emphasis on better policy coordination and the use of policy appraisal to assess the consequences of policies for health. A cross-departmental ministerial committee, supported by a group of officials drawn from across government departments, was established to oversee the implementation, monitoring and development of the strategy for England and to coordinate UK-wide issues affecting health. Health authorities were expected to collaborate with other agencies to tackle key national as well as locally set priorities. Task forces – drawn from government, the NHS, business and academia – developed coordinated programmes of action on specific issues, to promote interagency cooperation and ensure effective implementation. In addition, the government promoted the idea of 'healthy alliances' between different agencies at local level, including the NHS, local government and other local public services, the voluntary sector, employers and the media. A number of settings were identified as examples of where such alliances could develop: hospi-tals, schools, prisons, homes, workplaces and environments (DH, 1993).

An evaluation of the HOTN strategy, commissioned by the incoming New Labour government (DH, 1998a), found that although the policy had an impor-tant symbolic value, emphasizing the importance of public health and health promotion, it failed to galvanize sufficiently the NHS and other organizations.

Public health remained a low priority for health authorities and their partners. There were three key problems, all relating to failures to coordinate policy and promote collaboration. First, efforts to promote collaboration within central government failed. Other government departments did not prioritize health, and there was a failure to coordinate initiatives across government. The ministerial committee on public health was inactive. Interdepartmental conflict was evident. But the problem was as much a failure of health leadership as poor coordination. Even the Department of Health and the NHS failed to give public health sufficient priority, reflected in the perception by NHS managers and health authorities that health targets were secondary to those relating to finance and healthcare services.

Second, much more could have been done to strengthen partnership working at local level. HOTN failed to engage local authorities, which perceived it as an NHS initiative. This was reinforced by targets that focused heavily on disease and risk factors rather than social, economic and environmental factors affecting health. There was no attempt to overcome well-known difficulties, evident in other areas where collaboration was needed (such as health and social care), in that the NHS and local government had different agendas, incentives and cultures. The ownership of HOTN might have been extended more effectively to the voluntary sector and other agencies. Moreover, additional resources could have been provided to support collaborative working. Performance management systems in the NHS, local government and other public services could have been reshaped to acknowledge the importance of the public health agenda. More radically, some advocated the establishment of dedicated public health partnership bodies at local level (Public Health Alliance, 1988).

Third, HOTN was at somewhat at odds with other aspects of government health policy, such as the creation of an internal market that divided NHS bodies into commissioners and service providers (Cm 555, 1989). This division was blamed for the fragmentation of public health expertise and practice (Flynn et al., 1996; Nettleton and Burrows, 1997). Furthermore, while commissioning had the potential to shift NHS resources into public health and promote collaboration by making service providers more responsive to budget holders, this proved an optimistic view. Prevention and health promotion services lacked the political profile and clout of healthcare services and lost out accordingly. Moreover, the decision to place a significant proportion of the NHS budget in the hands of GPs meant that commissioning was strongly oriented towards healthcare for individual patients rather than public health priorities (DH, 1998a). GPs were generally poor at working in partnership with other agencies on service provision, and this impeded collaboration (Taylor et al., 1998; Moon and North, 2000).

Developments up to the present day

From the late 1990s onwards, governments redoubled their efforts to strengthen collaboration and partnership working in public health. These efforts are considered in detail in later chapters. This historical account has identified a number of key themes, useful as a means of contextualizing recent and current developments in this field. First, issues of partnership and collaboration are long-standing and in some respects as old as public health itself. Second, the location and distribution of responsibilities across institutions at various levels of governance has often been suboptimal from a public health perspective. Third, public health considerations have often lost out to other priorities, such as the quest for profits and administrative or professional claims over territory. Fourth, effective collaboration on public health matters often requires active intervention – it rarely happens by chance – and is likely to absorb much political effort and resources.

Exploring and understanding partnerships

The final part of this chapter focuses upon the how best to approach the study of partnerships and, in so doing, clarifies key terms and concepts. The starting point is with key concepts and terminology. This is followed by an examination of the rationale for partnerships and the factors that encourage their adoption. Finally, the evaluation and effectiveness of partnerships is discussed.

Partnerships

According to Ling (2000, p. 82), the literature on partnerships is characterized by 'methodological anarchy and definitional chaos', while the Institute for Public Policy Research (2001, p. 39) accepted that 'there is not, and probably never will be, a universally accepted definition of partnership'. The wider literature reflects these comments (Balloch and Taylor, 2001; Glendinning et al., 2002; Sullivan and Skelcher, 2002; Dowling et al., 2004; Glasby and Dickinson, 2008).

The term 'partnership' is used rather loosely and is often employed as a rhetorical 'ideal' to galvanize agencies to work together. The term is rarely defined, and even when it is, this tends to be based on general descriptive features. For example, Powell and Glendinning (2002, p. 3) defined partnership as 'the involvement of at least two agents or agencies with at least some common interests or interdependencies; and would also probably require a relationship between them that involves a degree of trust, equality or reciprocity'. The Audit Commission (1998, p. 8) defined it as a joint working arrangement in which partners are otherwise independent bodies, agree to cooperate to achieve a common goal, create a new organizational structure or process to achieve this goal, plan and implement a joint programme, and share relevant information, risks and rewards. Similarly, Sullivan and Skelcher (2002) identified partnerships by their key activities: sharing responsibility for assessing the need for action, determining the type of action to be undertaken and agreeing implementation; negotiating between people from diverse agencies; a commitment to working beyond the short term; aiming to secure the delivery of benefits or added value that could not have been achieved by a single agency acting on its own; and involving a formal articulation of purpose and plan to bind partners together.

Confusion arises from the many different kinds of partnership that exist, which makes generalization difficult if not impossible. Partnerships vary according to the kind of participant involved. There are partnerships between public sector bodies, between government and private sector or voluntary bodies, between non-government bodies, and between professional groups. Partnerships are also used to describe a relationship between government and society, or with particular social groups. In addition, there is much variation in specific partnership arrangements. Some are highly formalized, while others are very informal. The style of partnership working is far from uniform. The governance of partnerships can vary. They may differ according to their degree of inclusiveness. Partnerships can be contrasted in the degree of voluntarism and autonomy they allow to participants. In addition, there can be a variation in partnership arrangements between different policy areas, again making it difficult to generalize. Complicating matters further, the characteristics of a partnership are not necessarily fixed over time (Lowndes and Skelcher, 1998), evolving as a result of internal factors or external factors such as policy, legislation and the allocation of resources.

The language used to describe partnership arrangements is imprecise (Huxham, 2003; Wildridge et al., 2008). As Dowling et al. (2004) observed, terms such as collaboration, cooperation, coordination, coalition, joint working, alliances, and so on, are often used interchangeably. However, there are concerns that these terms are not identical, but have different meanings and nuances. Gray (1989, p. 5) made a distinction between collaboration (defined as 'a process through which parties who see different aspects of a problem can constructively explore their differences and search for solutions that go beyond their own limited vision of what is possible'), coordination (a more formal and institutionalized approach than collaboration) and cooperation (a looser and less formal way of producing reciprocity than collaboration).

Nonetheless, there remains wide disagreement on the meaning of these and other terms. Figure 1.1 attempts to clarify the meaning of these terms, although it is important to note that the field is contested.

Rather than arguing endlessly over precise meanings, it is perhaps better to acknowledge the diversity of partnership arrangements. Perhaps the best way of dealing with this complexity is to view partnership as an activity that can take place in many different settings, at various levels, with different kinds of participants (Sullivan and Skelcher, 2002). Partnerships can be analysed as a set of institutions, processes and relationships that survive beyond the immediate period, that have been established to achieve common or mutual aims, and in which the participants take some responsibility for achieving these aims.

The literature on public health and well-being partnerships reflects the problems of terminology found in the wider partnership literature. Terms such as 'collaboration', 'partnerships' and 'alliances' are often used interchangeably, and few attempts have been made to define these concepts. However, a useful definition of healthy alliances was devised by Powell (cited by Funnell et al., 1995, p. 78): 'a partnership of organizations and/or individuals to enable people to increase control over and to improve health and wellbeing, emotionally, physically, mentally, socially and environmentally.' Roussos and Fawcett (2000, p. 369) meanwhile defined collaborative partnerships in public health as 'people and organizations from multiple sectors working together in common purpose', their aim being to

Figure 1.1	The lexicon of partnership

Alliance
An arrangement between two or more parties for a common purpose

Coalition
A temporary arrangement between two or more parties for a common purpose

Collaboration
A process established by two or more parties to explore and establish working arrangements for a common purpose

Cooperation
An informal agreement between two or more parties to work together for a common purpose

Coordination
A highly formalised or institutional arrangement between two or more parties to work together for a common purpose

Co-production
A process between two or more parties (usually state and private/voluntary agencies or individuals) that produces a defined output or outcome

Interdisciplinary/multidisciplinary working
Arrangements to work together between people from different disciplines and/or bodies of subject expertise

Interorganizational working
Arrangements to work together between two or more organizations

Interprofessional working
Arrangements to work together between two or more professional groups

Intersectoral/multisectoral working
Arrangements to work together across different arenas and sectors (e.g. housing, education and health)

Joined-up government
Different parts of government working together for a common purpose

Joint action
Clearly defined actions to address a common purpose, agreed by two or more parties

Joint working
Working arrangements agreed between two or more parties

Multiagency/interagency working
Arrangements between different agencies (including non-government bodies) to work together

Networks and networking
Looser forms of communication, knowledge sharing and information exchange between a large number of parties

Partnership
Where two or more parties commit to work together for a common purpose

'attempt to improve conditions and outcomes related to the health and wellbeing of entire communities'. Building on these definitions, and explicitly acknowledging the national, international as well as local dimensions of collaboration, this book adopts a broad working definition of public health partnerships, as follows:

> Public health and well-being partnerships comprise a range of collaborative working arrangements, institutions and processes, involving organizations and individuals, that seek to improve the health and well-being of individuals and communities at various levels, nationally, locally and globally.

Partnerships and governance

Partnership working, collaboration and 'joined-up' approaches to public policy problems have been linked to 'governance' (Rhodes, 1997; Stoker, 1998; Pierre and Peters, 2000; Newman, 2001; Richards and Smith, 2002; Kooiman, 2003). While the term 'governance' is itself contested, most would agree that it refers to the development of particular ways of governing that involve institutions and actors which would previously have been considered as beyond the scope of government. It is argued that changes in the political environment (declining faith in government and the welfare state and the rise of neoliberalism) and in society at large (greater diversity, consumerism, voluntarism and individualism) as well as other factors (such as globalization and technology) have challenged existing forms of hierarchical government and blurred boundaries between the public and private sectors. Meanwhile, nation states have ceded power and authority to other tiers of government (supranational institutions and devolved governments, for example) and to quasi-governmental agencies and private corporations. This 'hollowing out' of the state (Rhodes, 1997) led to the development of forms of governance in which governing is undertaken increasingly through steering, coordination and regulation, bringing 'non-governmental actors' more closely into processes of policy-making and implementation. Policy networks and partnership arrangements, inhabited by government and non-government organizations, have therefore become key arenas of governance (Skelcher, 2000; Newman, 2001).

As indicated, there are different perspectives on governance (see Newman, 2001, and Richards and Smith, 2002, for a further discussion). Some emphasize its radicalism and novelty, and the scope for democratization and dispersal of power. Others are more sceptical, highlighting continuities between the era of 'government' and that of 'governance', and some are very critical of the concept of governance and its application. Indeed, there have been a number of challenges to the idea of governance both as an empirical reality and as a normative ideal. Policy networks and partnership working are not entirely new phenomena and precede the changes in government and the political environment mentioned above (Newman, 2001; Richards and Smith, 2002). Moreover, forms of networked governance, including partnerships, may in fact be hierarchy by another name, as government participants continue and even extend their pre-eminence within these structures (Newman, 2001; Whitehead, 2007; Miller and

Rose, 2008; Davies, 2011; Fenwick et al., 2012). In other words, the capacity of government to exert power and authority may be enhanced rather than diminished by these arrangements.

The rationale for partnerships is rooted in the more sanguine view of governance, which is in turn based on a rational response to problems of public policy-making (Challis et al., 1988; Audit Commission, 1998; Lowndes and Skelcher, 1998; Miller and Ahmad, 2000; Sullivan and Skelcher, 2002; Boydell et al., 2008). This has several aspects. First, partnerships are seen as a response to the challenges of difficult or 'wicked' issues (Rittel and Webber, 1973; Clarke and Stewart, 1997). Such issues are characterized by difficulties of definition and problems of ascertaining causality. They involve complex interdependencies and are difficult if not impossible for agencies to tackle alone. It is believed that such problems are increasingly common as society becomes more complex. As a result, agencies must work more closely together than hitherto.

Second, and related to this, it is argued that agencies must work together more effectively in order to overcome the 'silo mentality' that is said to characterize modern government at all levels. The modern setting therefore requires new forms of governance, including partnership working, to improve the response to social problems (Kooiman, 2003).

Third, specific advantages arising from partnerships have been identified (Audit Commission, 1998). Transaction costs may be reduced through partnership working. Further efficiencies and service improvements may be derived, due for example to the avoidance of duplication and suboptimal 'cost-shunting' (the shifting of problems and costs onto other agencies). It is possible that partnerships may bring a better mutual understanding of problems, thus providing a springboard for innovation. Benefits may also arise from the pooling of resources, skills and expertise and the sharing of information.

Finally, where the partnership approach is extended to the wider community, voluntary organizations and the private sector, it can in theory bridge the gap between government and the governed, harness social resources and provide greater responsiveness to the needs and preferences of citizens and to business interests.

These advantages can be summarised as 'collaborative advantage'. This is the sum total of gains from collaboration, or 'something has to be achieved that could not have been attained by any of the organizations acting alone' (Huxham, 2003, p. 403). Similarly, Lasker et al. (2001, p. 184) have highlighted the importance of 'partnership synergy', which is more than the mere exchange of resources: 'By combining the individual perspectives, resources and skills of the partners, the group creates something new and valuable together – a whole that is greater than the sum of its individual parts.'

Although partnership working is widely acknowledged as a beneficial approach, one should not accept it uncritically. The literature on collaboration warns of the dangers of making assumptions about rationale and benefits. Challis et al. (1988), in a landmark study of joint approaches to social policy, pointed out two main traditions within the debate about interagency collaboration, each based on different normative values and assumptions. The optimistic tradition is based on a rational, top-down approach to decision-making, a belief in technical competence and planning, an assumption that collaboration will further the public good, and a desire for unification, order and harmony. In contrast, the pessimistic approach disputes that there is a harmony of needs and focuses instead on the divergent interests. It is based on a belief that action to coordinate policy is not necessarily based on a desire to maximize the public good (although, rhetorically, this is often deployed as a justification). This less sanguine approach is sceptical about the ability of government to manage complex systems in a top-down way. It highlights problems of information and communication and the multifaceted nature of policy (seeing it as a complex interactive process with many streams rather than a single authoritative blueprint). The pessimistic approach does not entirely rule out the possibility of collaboration, however, but rejects top-down rational planning, suggesting that a better approach would be to facilitate bargaining and exchange between the different organizations concerned.

Notably, in their study, Challis et al. (1998) found both approaches to be flawed. Hence, they devised a third approach, which incorporated aspects of each. This 'planned bargaining model' acknowledged that government had a legitimate role in designing the institutional architecture but that it must incorporate insights into how people and organizations behave. In particular, it must be designed in such a way that it provides incentives for participants to collaborate, facilitates a strong representation of clients' interests, and provides opportunities to evaluate and learn from experience.

One of the key lessons from this and other work on partnership and collaboration (Wilkinson and Appleby, 1999; Rummery, 2002; Huxham, 2003; Jones and Stewart, 2009) is that efforts to improve matters may have unforeseen or adverse consequences. There are several potential problems here:

■ Partnership is not necessarily a zero-sum game. Some organizations and individuals may be disadvantaged by partnership arrangements, while others gain.
■ Whereas partnership may produce benefits, especially for clients, and may lead to efficiency gains for organizations, it also consumes resources in terms of monetary and opportunity costs (for example, the additional staff time required to engage in partnership structures and processes).
■ Partnership working usually involves coercion and the establishment of regulatory frameworks and rules. This tends to increase the power of higher tier authorities, in particular central government. It also tends to centralize power within central government itself. Authoritarian and coercive forms of partnership working may actually damage genuine efforts to build partnerships by preventing the 'horizontal' sharing of mutually beneficial goals. By becoming an end in itself, top-down partnership working may sap existing energies that might otherwise have mobilized 'bottom-up' partnership activity.
■ Partnership working can weaken political, professional and financial accountability and responsibility. As an increasing number of decisions are made by partnership bodies, it is possible for those agencies directly accountable for specific services to evade responsibility for joint services. This undermines accountability, unless a way is found to hold the partnership body to account. Even then, individual agencies may hide behind collective responsibility,

blaming the partnership body for any failings. Collective responsibility may in practice enable abdication of responsibility.

■ Partnership working may be undertaken for many different reasons. However, authorities and agencies may disguise their main reasons for partnership working, highlighting instead those that are more attractive and appealing. For example, the ability to meet clients' needs more effectively might be given as the principal justification for partnership working, whereas the real aim may be the reduction of overall expenditure on services across different agencies.

The point is that an understandable desire for a more rational system of governance and service provision, and better outcomes from policy and services, must not distract from the potential shortcomings of partnership working, such as weakened accountability, centralization, financial and other costs, and adverse distributional effects.

Factors encouraging partnership working

Partnership working has grown and developed for three main reasons. First, it has been actively endorsed and promoted by central government. Second, it has been closely associated to several key international policy agendas. Third, it was able to develop out of existing relationships and processes, at regional, local and grass-roots levels.

For many years, central government has promoted partnerships, across a number of policy areas. During the late 1960s, for example, area-based initiatives sought to address deep-rooted social problems by bringing together various agencies and involving local communities (Foley and Martin, 2000). In the 1970s, as noted earlier, joint planning and financing arrangements were introduced to develop health and social care services. This was in the context of wider efforts by central government to produce a joint approach to social policy (Challis et al., 1988). In the 1980s and 1990s, under the Conservative governments of Thatcher and Major, partnerships were encouraged in a number of areas, including, once again, regeneration programmes, health and social care, and, under Major, public health. During this period, the private sector was heralded as a provider of welfare services and a key contributor to policy outcomes. Consequently, partnerships between public and private sectors were encouraged. The voluntary sector was also increasingly acknowledged as a partner in social policy.

Under New Labour, however, there was a 'step-change' (Miller and Ahmad, 2000). 'Joined-up government' became a key policy theme (Cm 4310, 1999; Williams, 1999; Performance and Innovation Unit, 2000). References to this and to partnership working appeared in policy documents on health, social care, child welfare, education, crime and regeneration (Balloch and Taylor, 2001; Glendinning et al., 2002; Sullivan and Skelcher, 2002). There was also a shift in focus away from merely encouraging partnerships towards an expectation that they would be the norm and, increasingly, mandatory (Newman, 2001). Meanwhile, there were continuing pressures to extend partnership to stakeholders outside the public sector, such as the private, voluntary and community sectors. There was also a stronger focus on public participation, patient and user involvement, and partnership with communities. The increasing attention given to partnership working by the Blair government was due to a variety of factors (Newman, 2001; Clarke and Glendinning, 2002).

The desire for a more collaborative approach was articulated as a key New Labour policy theme linked to the Third Way (Driver and Martell, 2002; Ludlam and Smith, 2004; Whitehead, 2007; Davies, 2009). However, although partnerships reflected communitarian and Third Way notions of inclusion and active citizenship (Etzioni, 1993; Tam, 1998), it is evident that this approach was not entirely new, having been pursued to some extent by previous Labour and Conservative governments. Furthermore, although New Labour perhaps attempted to deploy partnerships more explicitly than its predecessor in policy development and implementation, this was as much due to the push of potential partners for recognition as to the pull of government to acknowledge and include them. What was perhaps different about New Labour was that the rhetoric of partnerships was much more prominent than previously. In addition, partnership became a much more explicit tool of central control and performance management than before.

Other factors, emerging in the mid-1980s and early 1990s and related to international policy agendas, also created favourable conditions for the expansion of partnership working. These included LA21, Health for All and Healthy Cities, mentioned above. In addition, European Union (EU) programmes emphasized the need for agencies (at both EU and member state level) to work together on environmental and health issues.

In addition, partnerships developed from the bottom up. Local individuals and organizations, frustrated at failure to make progress, forged relationships with others to seek solutions to difficult problems. In some cases, partnerships developed out of the efforts of a particular individual or a small group. Such 'champions' are often service managers or professionals (Hudson, 1995; Hudson et al., 1997). Another relevant concept is the 'boundary-spanner' (Williams, 2011), actors whose primary job involves managing within multiorganizational and multisectoral arenas. The role of champions and boundary-spanners indicates the importance of local management and professional cultures in improving services through partnership. It is also recognized that individuals based in voluntary or community sector organizations can play important roles in building and maintaining local partnerships. This suggests that social capital, the networks, norms and trust that exist to a lesser or greater extent in communities (see Box 5.1), is important in promoting and developing partnership working and service improvement.

Evaluating partnerships: evidence and effectiveness

A tendency to assume rather than evaluate the effectiveness of partnerships has been noted (Powell and Glendinning, 2002; Hunter et al., 2011). Even where evaluation has taken place, most studies focus on process rather than outcomes (Cameron and Lart, 2003). Process evaluation is not, however, irrelevant. It can detect important changes in the capacity of governing organizations and their partners to understand and respond to complex environments and social problems

(Boydell et al., 2008). Partnership working may contribute greatly to such 'intangible assets', which in the longer term may improve outcomes. Even so, the evidence gap regarding outcomes must be addressed (Dowling et al., 2004; Smith, K. et al., 2009; Perkins et al., 2010), notwithstanding the considerable methodological difficulties involved (Kreuter et al., 2000; El Ansari et al., 2001).

There are particular difficulties in demonstrating that health and well-being outcomes are due to partnership-based interventions. Evidence generated tends to compare unfavourably with that from clinical trials and laboratory-based research, particularly from the perspective of the dominant medical research establishment. Guidelines have been produced on the design of such studies (Craig et al., 2008). However, these have been criticised for failing to reflect the realities of community-based interventions, such as the difficulties of standardizing contexts and interventions, separating control and intervention groups, and maintaining a stable research environment for the duration of the study (Mackenzie et al., 2010). That said, many of the problems of evaluation in the field of partnership-based interventions can be attributed to poor evaluation and, in some cases, a complete failure to evaluate (Health Committee, 2009). Not surprising then that a systematic review found little evidence of the direct effects of public health partnerships (Smith, K. et al., 2009; Perkins et al., 2010). Where positive outcomes were found, it was difficult to attribute them to partnership working for various reasons: partnership working was rarely defined, the interventions did not rely solely on partnership working but overlapped with similar interventions, or the public health aims shifted during the lifetime of the intervention.

Although empirical work on partnerships is regarded as generating insufficient evidence on their effectiveness, the current evidence base does give some indication of their potential value, the problems they face and the factors that appear to enhance or limit their effectiveness.

The problems of partnership

The literature on partnerships generally is heavily oriented towards the identification and resolution of problems. Indeed, as Huxham (2003) observed, 'collaborative inertia' is common. Partnerships often struggle to deliver outcomes, and when they do 'pain and hard grind' is involved (Huxham, 2003, p. 403). There are many reasons why partnerships fall short of their aspirations (see, for example, Audit Commission, 1998, 2005; Hudson and Hardy, 2002; Cameron and Lart, 2003; Glasby and Dickinson, 2008; Wistow, 2012). Sometimes the objectives are unclear. A common vision may be lacking. Underlying conflicts of interest may exist. There could be major organizational and cultural differences between partner organizations. This can be underpinned by different professional cultures, arising from partner organizations employing professional groups, each with their own narrow perspective. In some cases, formal arrangements may impede effective partnership working on the ground. Planning and management systems and processes of partner agencies may be at variance. Difficulties may arise from the lack of common geographical boundaries (or co-terminosity). Constant reorganization and structural reform may further disrupt partnership working (Cameron and Lart, 2003). There may be poor leadership or weak commitment from the partners and their senior decision-makers. There could be a history of low trust between participants, which is difficult to overcome. Accountability arrangements may be inadequate. Agencies may be unwilling or unable to share information with each other. There might be a failure to evaluate the impact of the partnership and learn from past successes and failures. Partnership working may also fail due to underresourcing. Other financial obstacles include different budgeting practices and incompatible budget cycles. Problems can also occur due to differences in perceived legitimacy between the participating agencies. A further issue encountered is that higher tier authorities may themselves not be working collaboratively, and this compounds difficulties in partnership working at lower levels. Another problem is that expectations about partnerships are often set unrealistically high (Kreuter et al., 2000).

Improving partnership working

On a more positive note, some have identified 'essential features' that partnerships must possess in order to succeed. These are based on observations and experience of partnership working, usually derived from case studies. Frye and Webb (2002) highlighted the following: the inclusion of all relevant bodies, a high level of trust, motivation by a common vision, clear objectives, collaboration based on collective responsibility and continued support from key sponsors. In addition, they argued that partnerships require flexibility, long-term funding and mechanisms to resolve conflict. Other studies and reviews (see, for example, Butterfoss et al., 1993; Audit Commission, 1998; Roussos and Fawcett, 2000; Mattesich et al., 2001; Sullivan and Skelcher, 2002; Weiss et al., 2002; Cameron and Lart, 2003; Dowling et al., 2004; Daley, 2008; Porter et al., 2008; Perkins et al., 2010) identify similar characteristics linked to success: trust, a clearly agreed purpose, a common vision, leadership and accountability, longevity of the partnership, a previous history of good collaboration, good communication, structural incentives, social capital and socioeconomic context. Some identify proximity (for example, the co-location of workers from different agencies) and joint training and team-building as effective in forging partnerships and making them work (Cameron and Lart, 2003).

These various criteria have been incorporated into models and frameworks of partnership working, which form the basis of evaluation and improvement. For example, Hudson and Hardy (2002; see also Hardy et al., 2000) devised a partnership assessment tool for health and social care (which has since been applied to other areas), based on six principles of successful partnerships:

- recognition and acceptance of the need for partnership;
- clarity and realism of purpose;
- commitment and ownership;
- development and maintenance of trust;
- clear and robust partnership arrangements;
- monitoring, measurement and learning.

A generic approach was taken by Moss-Kanter (1994), who identified the fundamental need of partners to shift from consideration of their own narrow perspective to a collective approach. This was characterized as the eight 'I's that make successful 'we's:

- *Individual excellence* – partners have something of value to contribute and are good at their core business.
- *Importance* – partners share major strategic objectives and want the partnership to work.
- *Interdependence* – the partners need each other and have complementary skills. They cannot do separately what they can achieve together.
- *Investment* – partners are willing to invest long term and are willing to commit resources such as time, people and money.
- *Information* – partners are willing to share information with each other, and there is an open relationship between them.
- *Integration* – partners develop linkages and shared ways of operating.
- *Institutionalization* – the relationship is given formal status with clear responsibilities and decision-making processes.
- *Integrity* – partners behave in an honourable way, build trust and do not undermine each other.

Moss-Kanter sees relationships in dynamic rather than static terms. In her view, partnerships, like personal relationships, can pass through different stages. Each stage has a particular character and involves different types of activities. In the 'early days', there is some compatibility and attraction and exploration of mutual interests. This is superseded by a 'going steady' period, where future possibilities are examined and plans developed. As 'partnerships become real', ideas are discovered about what needs to be done to address common needs. There is then a 'settling down' period where mechanisms are developed for producing compromise and action. Finally, the partners 'grow old together', changing internally as a result of accommodating the ongoing partnership. Like personal relationships, some partnerships will flourish and survive long term, while others will not get beyond the early stages (and some may end in divorce!).

In addition to generic models of partnership working, public health-specific models have been devised. For example, Nutbeam (1994) identified several 'preconditions' to increase the prospects of intersectoral partnerships: clear definition of the issue, community support and understanding of the issue, and mutual respect between partners. In addition, he identified additional factors that could help to improve the outcomes of partnerships once established: providing leadership, defining the task clearly, delineating roles and responsibilities, and providing a recognizable 'exit point', recognizing that new alliances may need to be formed and old partnerships ended as issues evolve.

The WHO (2010a) identified a number of criteria against which public health partnerships could be assessed and which might indicate ways of improving partnerships. These were:

- clear added value for public health (such as mobilization of partners, knowledge and resources);

- clear goals in line with public health priorities (of WHO), within a realistic time frame;
- guidance by technical norms and standards (of WHO);
- support of national development objectives;
- ensuring an appropriate and adequate participation of stakeholders;
- a clear role for partners;
- evaluation of transaction costs, benefits and risks;
- the pursuit of public health goals taking precedence over special interests of the participants, with mechanisms to identify and manage conflicts of interest;
- the structure of the partnership corresponding to the proposed functions (i.e. less formal structures for looser forms of cooperation);
- independent external evaluation and/or self-monitoring mechanisms.

Also pertinent here is the *Adelaide Statement on Health in All Policies* (WHO and Government of South Australia, 2010) which sets out a number of factors that enhance the integration of health, equity and well-being in policies. These include: a clear mandate to make joined-up working an imperative; systematic processes that take account of interactions across sectors; mediation across different interests; accountability, transparency and participatory processes; engagement with stakeholders outside government; and practical cross-sector initiatives to build partnerships and trust. In addition, the statement identified a host of tools and instruments that could contribute to 'health in all policies', including interministerial and interdepartmental committees, cross-section action teams, integrated budgets, cross-cutting information and evaluation systems, joined-up workforce development, community consultation, impact assessments, legislative frameworks, health lens analysis and partnership platforms. A set of key drivers was also highlighted, including: creating strong partnerships that recognize mutual interests and share targets; building a 'whole of government' commitment by engaging the head of government, Cabinet and Parliament as well as the administrative leadership; developing strong high-level policy processes; embedding responsibilities into government's overall strategies, goals and targets; ensuring joint decision-making and accountability for outcomes; enabling openness and full consultative approaches to encourage the endorsement of stakeholders and advocacy; encouraging experimentation and innovation; pooling intellectual resources, integrating research and sharing wisdom; and providing feedback mechanisms so that progress can be evaluated and monitored at the highest level.

Evaluation criteria were devised as part of a tool for planning, evaluating and developing healthy alliances (Funnell et al., 1995). This work identified two types of indicator: processes and outputs. Process indicators included commitment (goals and resources), community participation (liaison with community, empowerment), communication (sharing information, accessibility of programmes), joint working (strategies, action plans and flexible responses to changing needs), and accountability (shared responsibility for outcomes and evaluation). Outputs included: policy change, changes in services and the environment, skills development, publicity, contact (with the public and service users) and knowledge, attitude and behaviour change. Another approach by Douglas (1998; building on work by Powell, 1992) formulated a three-dimensional framework of assessment that reflected future potential as well as past achievement: (1) assessing potential (past and present relationships, core purposes and priorities, and the nature and extent of collaboration); (2) joint working (resource exchange and flexibility, extent of user/patient/community involvement, and the nature of leadership and coordinated activity); and (3) assessing achievement (outcomes or health gains achieved, service gains or changes, and organizational learning).

Such frameworks help us to think about the aims and purpose of partnerships and provide a useful tool for evaluation, analysis and improvement. In this context, Hudson (1987) provides a simple and useful classification for thinking about how collaboration and partnership can be fostered. Essentially, there are three main approaches. First, mutual cooperation can be encouraged. Second, incentives can be provided. Third, cooperation can be mandated by higher tier authorities. In practice, one or more of these strategies may be adopted.

Analysing partnerships

This book seeks to analyse partnerships in the field of public health and well-being. It looks at how partnerships have emerged and how they have operated in practice. It examines their achievements and shortcomings, as well as possible ways of enhancing the former and overcoming the latter. It is certainly not a manual on how to improve partnership working, but it may stimulate reflection on the dilemmas and problems of working together for public health and well-being.

The structure of this book reflects the different dimensions of partnership, in particular that partnership occurs at different levels of government (Rhodes, 1997; Bache and Flinders, 2004). In Chapter 2, partnerships at the global and international level are discussed, including the experience of other countries. Chapter 3 explores the record of New Labour in promoting partnerships between different public sector agencies, such as the NHS and local government. Chapter 4 explores the policies of the Cameron Coalition government and their potential impact on partnerships. Chapter 5 examines partnerships between government agencies and the public and service users, while Chapter 6 focuses on the relationship between government and the voluntary sector. The relationship between the public sector and private 'for-profit' sector is explored in Chapter 7, and Chapter 8 brings together the key themes and reflects on the future of partnerships in public health and well-being in the UK.

2 Partnerships at the global and international level

Introduction

Global and international factors have provided a rationale for public health partnerships and have yielded important lessons for partnership working. Three key aspects are considered in this chapter. First are the global aspects of partnership, including initiatives undertaken by bodies such as the World Health Organization (WHO), and the processes that link global institutions and organizations. Second are the activities of European bodies, such as European Union (EU) institutions and the WHO European Regional Office. Third are the experiences of particular countries in establishing and developing partnership arrangements.

The global level

Although public health has tended to be a 'nationally-focused endeavour' (Collin and Lee, 2007, p. 105), it is acknowledged that significant causes of ill health transcend national borders. Cross-border threats to health are not entirely new, as the history of epidemics clearly shows (Berlinguer, 1999). Even so, there is a widespread belief that international threats to health are increasing and becoming more complex as a result of globalization (Labonte and Shrecker, 2004; Lee and Collin, 2005; Koivusalo, 2006) – the increasing interconnectedness of nations through finance, trade, politics, culture, technology and communication, which makes it ever more difficult for them to make decisions independently of others (Giddens, 1999; Held and McGrew, 2000).

The health consequences of globalization (see Yach and Bettcher, 1998a; Kickbusch and de Leeuw, 1999; Lee and Collin, 2005; Kickbusch and Seck, 2007) include:

■ the health consequences of global environmental threats such as climate change (for example, rising levels of infectious disease, a higher number of deaths from some cancers, heart and respiratory diseases, displacement of the population due to extreme weather events and rising sea levels, and the consequences of damage to ecological and agricultural systems; *Lancet* and UCL Institute for Global Health Commission, 2009);

- the spread of infectious disease (such as influenza) due to increased travel and trade;
- the growth of chronic diseases, such as obesity and smoking-related disease, due to the spread of Western consumer cultures and lifestyles;
- the health consequence of growing socioeconomic inequities, both within and between countries, as a result of the concentration of capital and economic power, privatization and the increasing use of markets to allocate resources;
- the health consequences of war, terrorism and population displacement caused by geopolitical and faith-based conflicts;
- the global trade in legal and illegal recreational drugs;
- the movement of health professionals from poorer to richer countries.

In addition, a number of problems are increasingly common to all countries of the world and therefore constitute a further set of 'global challenges'. These include the emergence of new diseases and variants of existing infectious diseases, resistant to treatment with existing drugs (for example, tuberculosis [TB] and new strains of influenza); growing elderly populations, which imply higher health service costs in the future; and the rising costs of healthcare systems (due partly to ageing populations and also to changing disease patterns and new technologies).

Consequently, 'global public health' has become a key concern (Stone, 2012). It has been defined as 'the collective ability to conduct healthy public policy at a global level through a network of public, private, non-governmental, national, regional and international organizations by regime formation' (Kickbusch and de Leeuw, 1999, p. 286). Collaboration and partnership at this level can help to realize important benefits for all countries. It is frequently argued that only by joining together in a common cause can countries meet global public health challenges (Yach and Bettcher, 1998b; Kickbusch and Seck, 2007; McKee, 2007; Stone, 2012). Moreover, health can be regarded as a 'global public good' (Kaul et al., 1999; Smith et al., 2003; Kickbusch and Seck, 2007) that can only be properly protected by collective action at the global level. More specifically, the benefits of partnership in global public health – which relate closely to the broader rationale for establishing partnerships (see Chapter 1) – can be delineated as follows. First, such partnerships may generate additional capacity to prevent and manage public health problems, such as the pooling of resources, access to bodies of expertise and the sharing of information. Second, they can facilitate shared experiences and learning about the nature of public health problems and how to respond to them. Third, they can contribute to synergy in public health, increasing the effectiveness of policy responses by identifying priorities, coordinating activities and reducing duplication of effort.

Several different types of partnership can be identified at the global level. First, there are partnerships between countries, which may lead to the creation of global processes or institutions. Second, there are partnerships between global institutions. Third, there are partnerships between global institutions and other interests, such as non-government organizations (NGOs) and private corporations. The main focus of this chapter is on the first two aspects (global public–private partnerships are examined in greater depth in Chapter 7).

Creating and maintaining global partnerships

WHO

The WHO, created as a specialist agency of the UN in 1948, has played a major role in building global public health partnerships. Its main functions are to provide scientific advice on health issues, to set international health standards, to prevent disease and to promote health (see Lee, 2009). The early work of the agency focused on infectious disease and included the formulation of international health regulations to require the notification of dangerous diseases (including plague, yellow fever and cholera). Subsequently, it sought to tackle infectious diseases through vaccination and education programmes. The important work of WHO in combatting infectious diseases continues, with the reformulation of the international health regulations extending its role in relation to outbreaks of disease while widening its remit to a greater range of threats to global health. However, it is also increasingly concerned with addressing the problem of chronic disease.

The WHO has placed great emphasis on 'healthy public policy' (Milio, 1986), and more recently 'health in all policies' (see Chapter 1), which calls on all sectors to contribute to the promotion of health within an integrated approach at all levels of government. The WHO has endorsed community engagement, ensuring that people participate in decisions and choices affecting their health. It has also urged that governments work closely with voluntary organizations and business. These themes provide a strong justification for partnership working as a means of raising standards of health and addressing causes of preventable illness and injury.

The WHO championed these important themes through a series of international conferences and declarations on health promotion. The Alma Ata conference, which produced a declaration on primary healthcare (WHO and UNICEF, 1978), identified intersectoral working and community involvement as key elements in achieving Health for All. The Ottawa Charter for Health Promotion (WHO, 1986) emphasized the importance of healthy public policy and the need to ensure that all sectors of government, business and society took responsibility for health. The Ottawa Charter also acknowledged the importance of communities undertaking collective action in the pursuit of health objectives. The 1988 Adelaide Declaration reiterated the importance of healthy public policy across all levels of government and called for new alliances of government and NGOs to provide impetus for health action (WHO, 1988). The Sundsvaal conference in 1991 focused on health and the environment, and again highlighted the importance of building alliances to promote health (WHO, 1991).

At Jakarta in 1997, the conference called for a strengthening of the capacity of communities to actively participate in health promotion, and emphasized the consolidation and expansion of partnerships for health between different sectors at all levels of government and society (WHO, 1997). It also called for the establishment of a global health promotion alliance and urged greater social responsibility for health among both the public and private sector. In Mexico in 2000, the themes of healthy public policy and intersectoral working were re-emphasized (WHO, 2000a). The Bangkok Charter of 2005 emphasized the importance of partnerships and alliances involving public and private bodies, NGOs, international organizations and civil society. It identified a key role for the health sector in developing policy and partnerships for health promotion, and reiterated the importance of empowering communities (WHO, 2005). It also called for integrated policy-making in government and international organizations, strong international agreements on health promotion and the development of effective mechanisms of global health governance.

At the most recent global health promotion conference, at Nairobi in 2009, a 'Call to Action' was produced (WHO, 2009). This aimed to close the implementation gap in health promotion through a series of recommendations that reprised familiar themes: the promotion of health in all sectors and settings, the extension of partnership working beyond the health sector, and the fostering of community participation and empowerment. More specifically, the call to action included recommendations to create intergovernmental regional bodies that would set a vision and agenda for health promotion. It also requested that WHO should be mandated to develop a global health promotion strategy and associated action plans. A further Health Promotion conference is to take place in 2013 in Helsinki, Finland, and will focus on promoting health through policy and partnership.

WHO strategies and policies have reflected these themes. The Health for All by the Year 2000 strategy (WHO, 1981), and its revised version, Health for All in the 21st Century (WHO, 1998a), encouraged healthy public policy, intersectoral working, partnerships and alliances to promote health, and community participation in health, through a series of recommendations. The Healthy Cities movement, launched by the WHO European Region, sought to put Health for All principles into practice in urban contexts (Ashton, 1992; Davies and Kelly, 1992), Its central aim was to improve the health of people by working across sectors. This was to be achieved through the creation of strong partnership mechanisms and community participation. By 1991, 30 cities had joined the programme across Europe, including the UK. This has since risen to over 600 municipalities worldwide.

The WHO's emphasis on collaboration and partnership has been reflected in the resolutions of its supreme decision-making body, the World Health Assembly. In 1998, Resolution 51.12 on health promotion urged member states to consolidate and expand partnerships in health and called for the formation of global health promotion networks at global, regional and local levels (WHO, 1998b). In addition, principles of global health leadership, coordination, participation and partnership were evident in the work of WHO commissions on key areas of policy. Examples include the WHO Commission on Macroeconomics and Health (2001) and the WHO Commission on Social Determinants of Health (2008).

The WHO has been proactive in setting out global initiatives, strategies and action plans on a range of public health issues. It has had a leading role in promoting global action on the prevention and control of non-communicable diseases (WHO, 2008a, 2008b; Box 2.1) and in strategies on food safety (WHO, 2002), diet, exercise and obesity (WHO, 2004) and alcohol (WHO, 2010b). The WHO also introduced a Framework Convention on Tobacco Control, which set out an international framework for regulation (WHO, 2003). In addition, it has explicitly backed partnership working initiatives involving the private sector, including programmes to tackle diseases such as HIV/AIDS, TB and malaria in developing countries (see Chapter 7).

Box 2.1	Global action on non-communicable disease

In the new millennium, efforts by the WHO to promote global action on specific health issues such as alcohol, tobacco, diet, physical activity and obesity began to build into a more comprehensive plan to address the causes of non-communicable disease (NCD). A global strategy on NCDs (WHO, 2008a) was developed, along with an action plan (WHO, 2008b) that emphasized the importance of intersectoral working and partnerships. Meanwhile, an attempt was made to raise the profile of NCDs within the UN as a whole. A ministerial declaration at the UN Economic and Social Council called for urgent action on NCDs (UN General Assembly, 2010). This led to a High Level Meeting of the General Assembly in September 2011, which produced a political declaration (UN General Assembly, 2012b). This acknowledged the need to address the prevention and control of NCDs using a multisectoral approach. Among the key commitments made by the UN was to set out a comprehensive monitoring framework, including indicators and targets. Subsequently, an overall target to reduce by 25 per cent premature mortality from NCDs by 2025 was agreed. Other agreed targets included reductions in smoking, physical inactivity and levels of salt in food. Discussion on other targets and indicators (for example, alcohol, obesity and fat intake) continues at the time of writing.

Another important area covered by the declaration related to partnership working, particularly to ensure that all sectors contribute to reducing the burden of NCDs. The WHO has been charged with task of reviewing options on how partnerships can be strengthened (UN General Assembly, 2012c; WHO, 2012a, 2012b). Meanwhile, the process of formulating a new action plan for NCDs began. An initial draft (October 2012) set out a range of proposals pertinent to partnership working, including a UN interagency task force, a stronger role for the WHO in coordinating NCD-related activity across UN agencies, and the inclusion of NCDs on other UN agendas (such as sustainable development) (WHO, 2012b). Recommendations for member states included the pursuit of a 'whole of government' approach with national, multisectoral NCD policies and a strategic plan, high-level interministerial committees under the head of state to ensure that health is incorporated in all policies, and a national coordinating unit. Member states would also be expected among other things to allocate resources to NCD control and prevention, and to establish a monitoring framework. These proposals are currently subject to further consultation and discussion.

Other global institutions

Although the WHO is an important leader and coordinator of global health initiatives, it operates in a crowded environment (Kickbusch and Seck, 2007; Lee, 2009). Other international agencies and supranational bodies have taken an increasing interest in health matters in recent decades. Business organizations have also played a much bigger role in public health programmes than hitherto. Meanwhile, other non-state bodies, such as charitable foundations and NGOs, have become more prominent, and new networks and partnerships have emerged (Lee and Collin, 2005; Prah Ruger and Yach, 2005).

Other UN bodies have taken a lead on health matters, reflected in the adoption of health objectives from the UN Millennium Development Goals, which include reducing child mortality, improving maternal health and tackling major diseases such as HIV/AIDS, TB and malaria (UN General Assembly, 2000). The UN has adopted overarching strategies (on women and children's health, for example) and other initiatives (for example, a Decade of Action on Road Safety). Health issues such as these have been considered by the UN General Assembly, which has recently focused on preventing non-communicable diseases (Box 2.1). UN bodies such as UNICEF, the Food and Agriculture Organization, UNESCO and the International Labour Organization have a major interest in health. Health is also relevant to other UN programmes, such as the Development Programme and Drugs Control Programme as well as other UN functions with regard to population, refugees, human rights and security (Lee and Collin, 2005).

Furthermore, health is pertinent to the UN's environmental agenda, and the work of the UN Environment Programme and the Intergovernmental Panel on Climate Change. As already noted, the health consequences of global warming, climate change and pollution are significant. Health is also an important consideration in sustainable development. Indeed, action on global environmental issues has been stimulated by health concerns, alongside other important considerations such as concerns for biodiversity, the depletion of natural resources and ecological systems (Elliott, 2004). Together, these pressures led to international cooperation on issues such as ozone layer depletion, greenhouse gas reduction, the management of waste products, and the regulation of chemicals and pollution. This included international agreements and protocols, for example on ozone-depleting chemicals, such as CFCs. Environmental concerns at the global level have also produced sustainable development initiatives, associated with the 'Earth Summit' held in Rio in 1992 (UN, 1993), which established health as a key element of the sustainable development agenda and encouraged cross-sector and collaborative working, notably in the form of Agenda 21 (and its local manifestation, LA21, mentioned in Chapter 1; Carter, 2007). In 2012, the Rio+20 Conference was held to assess progress since the Earth Summit. Health featured strongly in the final outcome document *The Future We Want* (UN, General Assembly, 2012a), which included a call for further international collaboration on global health, including action on the social determinants of health and on communicable and non-communicable disease, as well as coordinated action on health across different sectors.

The World Bank, an autonomous body within the UN system, has developed a much greater role in health in recent times (Prah Ruger, 2005). Initially established as a financial body to stimulate economic reconstruction in industrialized countries in the immediate postwar period, its primary function became the financing of long-term programmes in developing countries (Marshall, 2008). From the 1980s, the World Bank pursued neoliberal policies, such as free trade, public expenditure cuts and privatization, and required borrowing countries to adopt these policies. It was able to exert much influence over policies affecting social welfare and health, often with adverse consequences (Lee and Collin, 2005). More recently, the World Bank has focused more on health, nutrition, poverty reduction, building social capital through community development, and establishing partnerships between government, the private sector and NGOs to improve health. It also began to take a more enlightened role on certain aspects of trade and health, exemplified by its withdrawal of support for the tobacco trade. It has also recently called for action on other non-communicable diseases, which it sees as a threat to the health and economic security of many lower and middle-income countries (World Bank, 2011).

Another autonomous body, the International Monetary Fund (IMF), impacts on health and welfare through its lending policies for countries in need of financial support. Its influence is arguably wider as its loans are not confined to the developing world. IMF loans carry certain conditions that often involve reducing public spending on health and welfare or pursuing policies that create conditions for business and trade (such as privatization or tax cuts and other neoliberal policies), with adverse public health consequences (Stuckler and Basu, 2009). Notably, the IMF can influence other financial flows and investment through its regular reports on the state of individual economies.

Similarly, the World Trade Organization (WTO), although not a UN agency, has a huge impact on health through its judgements on international trade rules. Although the WTO ostensibly protects health, by setting out conditions where such considerations are permitted to outweigh free trade principles (World Trade Organization, 1994), it is believed that trade considerations are paramount (Lee et al., 2009; Smith, R. et al., 2009). There are, however, dissenting views. For example, Mitchell and Voon (2011) argue that although the WTO has restricted countries from implementing public health measures, there is sufficient scope to design effective measures that minimize the impact on trade. They also point out that there is considerable scope for using WTO rules to improve health (by challenging subsidies on unhealthy products, for example).

Other international economic bodies with a significant role in international health governance include the Organisation for Economic Co-operation and Development (OECD) and the World Economic Forum (WEF). The OECD's stated aims are to promote economic growth, standards of living and international trade through agreement, and its membership contains the main industrialized nations. Although it lacks the economic and financial power of the IMF, World Bank and WTO, it can exert a more subtle impact on domestic policies by facilitating agreements, undertaking research reports and comparing the performance of member states (Armingeon and Beyeler, 2004). The OECD has a health committee and has produced reports, focusing particularly on the comparative performance of healthcare systems. Its activities produce peer pressure for reform, especially on cost-effectiveness grounds. The OECD is seen as promoting neoliberal principles, although in perhaps a less overt way (de Vos et al., 2004).

Meanwhile, the declared aim of the WEF is to create a world-class corporate governance system by harnessing entrepreneurship in the public interest. It aims to become the foremost organization for leading global communities, achieving economic and social progress by bringing corporate expertise and resources to bear on the world's problems. More specifically, it seeks to build partnerships between business, policy-makers and NGOs, and places great emphasis on developing strategic insights through their interaction. The WEF has been active on health issues, establishing a global health initiative in 2002. This led to partnership programmes and activities in specific disease areas (HIV/AIDS, TB and malaria) targeting particular parts of the world (Africa, China and India). The WEF is regarded by critics as an elitist organization, bringing together senior business people and policy-makers, while lacking a vision of how to involve communities and the grass roots. It has also been criticized for its pro-business, developed country and neoliberal stance (Pigman, 2007).

Global forums

Health has also achieved prominence on the international agendas of high-level global political forums such as the G7, G8 and G20 (Labonte and Shrecker, 2004). For example, the G7 and G8 summits (which comprise the world's richest countries) have discussed a range of health-related issues including food security, climate change, HIV/AIDS and drugs. These have led to commitments on the reduction of global poverty and disease (notably AIDS, TB and malaria), and have supported action on maternal and child health, for example. The G20, which includes industrializing countries such as China and India, has also considered health issues, although it has yet to develop a clear role in this field (Batniji and Woods, 2009). Other groups of countries, such as the Commonwealth and the Caribbean Countries, have urged a stronger global response to public health problems, including non-communicable diseases, in recent years.

The interest of some global political forums and groups in health has often been prompted by concerns about security, especially since '9/11'. This means that health threats or risks are construed as risks to the economy, the food system or the state, with wide political consequences. This 'framing' of health issues is something of a double-edged sword (Wallace-Brown and Harman, 2011). On the one hand, the 'securitization' of health threats can be seen as a positive development raising the profile of health on high-level agendas. It can also lead to decisions and additional resources that may benefit global health. But it also is very limiting because it is believed to distort health priorities. Health issues are seen as important in terms of their security implications more than anything else. This can result in a focus on key threats or diseases rather than on improving health overall. It can lead to certain problems being exaggerated while others are neglected. It may also encourage a piecemeal, disjointed and inconsistent approach to health problems.

Problems with global health governance

Several problems have been identified with the current system of global health governance. First, it is argued that there is a lack of leadership and strategy (Gostin et al., 2010). The WHO has to some extent been eclipsed by other bodies and has been unable to exercise strong leadership, due to funding problems, political pressure from the most powerful capitalist states, conflicts of interest and organizational and management weakness (Yamey, 2002a, 2002b; Earle, 2007; Lee, 2009; Legge, 2012; WHO, 2012a, 2012b; Mackey and Liang, 2013). As a result, key priorities have not been fully addressed. Some argue that there has been an overemphasis on infectious disease at the expense of chronic illness (Ollila, 2005; McKee, 2007). Although infectious diseases such as TB, HIV/AIDS and malaria represent major threats to health and deserve to be among the global priorities, much less attention has been given until fairly recently to chronic illnesses, despite the threats they pose to developing and developed countries. Even though this imbalance is now being addressed, the emerging powers in global health governance (WEF, G7/8 and the majority of public–private partnerships) continue to focus heavily on infectious disease. Moreover, they adopt a narrow focus on technological solutions to these problems, rather than considering socioeconomic interventions and investment in healthcare systems.

Second, partly resulting from the lack of strong leadership, there has been a tendency for health issues to be outweighed by other considerations, such as trade and economic growth. The WHO and other health-focused bodies have struggled against the dominant philosophy of free trade and market liberalization. They have been outgunned by economic, trade and financial bodies such as the WTO, World Bank, WEF and IMF, the USA and other neoliberal states, and large multinational corporations (Lee and Collin, 2005; Ollila, 2005; McKee, 2007; Smith, R. et al., 2009; Legge, 2012). For example, although the WHO has raised the importance of health standards in trade agreements with the WTO, and has pressed for a more appropriate balance between trade and health issues at national level, economic and financial issues continue to predominate.

Third, the plurality of bodies involved in health issues makes it difficult to coordinate policies and programmes (Kickbusch and Payne, 2004; Kickbusch and Seck, 2007; Gostin et al., 2010; Mackey and Liang, 2013). This means that even when there is a strong consensus about how to tackle a particular problem, there is no clear command structure, as well as an absence of coordination mechanisms to ensure that policies are properly implemented. The tendency of global leaders to bypass existing systems and create new initiatives has exacerbated this situation. Related to this is the acknowledgement that different agendas with common concerns are rarely linked. Hence development, health and environment agendas have often identified similar threats and concerns, but there has been little effort to integrate them. In recent years, however, there has been greater awareness of how these issues are connected. For example, the WHO and the UN Environment Programme launched a joint initiative to link health and environment agendas (WHO/UNEP, 2011). There has also been a greater acknowledgement of the connection between health and development (see below), but much more must be done to bridge these agendas.

Fourth, there is weak accountability in global health governance (Kickbusch and Seck, 2007; Gostin et al., 2010). This is partly a problem of shared responsibilities. It is difficult to hold institutions to account when responsibilities are unclear and they can blame each other for shortcomings. It has been argued that such arrangements should incorporate democratic commitments and safeguards for the public interest (Pinet, 2003). This applies equally to global institutions as well. The democratic deficit in global governance must be addressed (Nye, 2001; Langmore and Fitzgerald, 2010). It is also argued that both global institutions and partnerships must acknowledge possible conflicts of interest. There have been concerns particularly about this in public–private partnerships (see Chapter 7 for a further discussion). Conflicts of interest are also found within global institutions themselves, including the WHO (Legge, 2012). For example, there has been disquiet about a lack of transparency about links between WHO advisors on pandemic flu and drug companies producing flu vaccines and antiviral medicines (Cohen and Carter, 2010).

Fifth, capacity has long been recognized as a problem at the international level (see, for example, WHO, 2005, 2009). In particular, there is a need for existing resources available for global action to be increased and harnessed more effectively, so that major health problems that require leadership and collaboration at this level can be appropriately addressed.

The above problems are widely acknowledged, and there is growing support for a stronger global approach to health, with better leadership and more effective systems of collaboration (Kickbusch and Payne, 2004; Collin and Lee, 2007; Crisp, 2007; Kickbusch and Seck, 2007; HM Government, 2008b; Gostin et al., 2010; Stone, 2012). Notably, the WHO is undergoing a process of reform to focus more on key priorities and improve its governance and management. Increasingly, as mentioned, the UN leadership has taken a role in strengthening commitments to health and improving coordination and collaboration on these matters. In recent years, there has also been action to acknowledge health as an important aspect of foreign policy. In 2007, the Foreign Ministers of seven countries – Norway, France, Thailand, South Africa, Brazil, Indonesia and Senegal – issued a joint ministerial declaration (the Oslo Declaration) to widen the scope of foreign policy to include health issues (Ministers of Foreign Affairs, 2007). This endorsed specific actions including strengthening leadership on health issues, particularly within the UN, building cooperation and collaboration among international agencies and bodies, reinforcing health as a key element in development and poverty reduction, and ensuring health has priority in decisions about trade issues.

Calls to widen the scope of foreign policy to include health promotion have also been endorsed by the EU (Council of the European Union, 2010). It has highlighted the need to take action to improve health at the global level, recognizing that health is a key element in poverty reduction, development and sustainable economic growth, and acknowledging that there must be stronger leadership on global health. The UN has responded by recognizing that a closer relationship between foreign policy and global health is necessary, and that international action to promote this is required (UN General Assembly, 2009a, 2012d). Meanwhile, there is greater pressure to keep global commitments under review. The UN Economic and Social Council, which has a mandate to review and coordinate the activities of UN bodies operating in the field of development, acquired greater powers in 2005. It is now able to undertake substantive reviews and examine coordination between development partners, which can be a catalyst for improving policy implementation and coordination. In 2009, a high-level ministerial review examined internationally agreed goals and commitments in regard to public health. This led to a series of recommendations, including that global health challenges require concerted and sustained action on the part of the international community, that foreign policy and global health must be more closely linked, that the international community must support states to address the social determinants of health, that cooperation must be strengthened to address new and unforeseen health threats, and that urgent action be taken on non-communicable disease (UN General Assembly, 2009b).

As Earle (2007) observed, globalization has not only created health problems, but also offered fresh opportunities to improve health. There is now greater awareness of global health problems and an acknowledgement of the changes needed to create stronger leadership and collaboration (see UN General Assembly, 2012c). Suggestions include strengthening the WHO within the UN system, increasing the powers of global health bodies, strengthening coordinating mechanisms, clarifying responsibilities and increasing accountability, transparency and democracy. One suggestion is to establish a UN Global Health Panel to lead and coordinate the activities of agencies, NGOs and other stakeholders in order to promote more effective global action on health (Mackey and Liang, 2013). Whether such initiatives are pursued, however, is another matter, and there are powerful ideological, national and corporate interests that are resistant to change.

Europe

The global emphasis on better coordination, intersectoral working and stronger partnerships has been reflected at the European level. Institutions have responded to the public health agenda and have developed strategies and collaborative approaches to these issues. This section focuses on the actions of the EU, the WHO European Region and the Council of Europe.

The EU

Under the Treaty of Rome (1957), which established the European Economic Community, health was reserved as a matter for member states. However, there was scope for health-related initiatives under the Treaty's social policy provisions. Furthermore, efforts to harmonize trade and employment regulation provided additional opportunities to introduce health and safety measures (Greer, 2009a; Nugent, 2010). The Single European Act (1987) further increased the scope for this. Although its principal aim was to stimulate competition and trade across the European Community by harmonizing regulations, health protection was a key criterion. This meant that in a number of areas (including food, tobacco and health and safety in the workplace), regulation was actually strengthened. Health regulations were also generated through the environmental agenda as a result of the Single European Act, which strengthened the European Community's powers in areas such as water quality, waste control, chemicals, noise pollution and air pollution, giving it significant influence over key instruments of environmental health policy.

The key problem, however, was that these powers lacked a strategic framework. The arrangement of health services to meet population needs was a jealously guarded function of member states. Although there were strong reasons for greater coordination of public health matters, member states feared losing their autonomy.

In 1992, the Maastricht Treaty, which created the EU, established a new responsibility for public health (Treaty on European Union, 1992). However, the new provision only enabled EU institutions to contribute towards protecting human health by encouraging cooperation and lending support to member states. Legislation was ruled out as a means of harmonization, but research, information and incentives (such as funding for projects) were permitted.

Following the Maastricht Treaty, the EU developed a framework for action, including the establishment of a network for the control and surveillance of communicable diseases. Specific programmes were formulated on cancer prevention, HIV/AIDS, drug addiction, health monitoring, pollution-related disease, injury prevention and rare diseases (Randall, 2001). Following, the BSE/Creutzfeldt–Jakob disease crisis, which revealed poor coordination between EU bodies and conflicts of interest between health and commerce, a new Directorate for Health and Consumer Protection was established within the European Commission (Box 2.2). Now known as the Directorate for Health and Consumers, this organization developed a stronger EU focus on public health. Even so, it is regarded as a relatively weak directorate, partly because of the greater strength of the economic, agriculture and trade directorates, and partly because important public health functions, such as those relating to environmental health and health and safety, remain in the hands of other directorates and agencies. The Amsterdam Treaty (European Union, 1997) further extended the powers of the EU, stating that 'a high level of human health protection shall be ensured in the definition and implementation of all community policies and activities.' Action could include measures to improve public health, prevent illness and disease, and obviate sources of danger to public health. It was agreed by member states that there should be greater cooperation in areas such as health monitoring and disease surveillance. But, again, harmonization of laws and regulations was not permitted.

Nonetheless, these developments provided a sufficient foundation for a public health strategy. A programme of work was set out for the period 2003–08, with several aims: to improve health information and knowledge for the development of public health, to enhance capacity to respond to health threats, and to address health determinants (Decision of the European Parliament and of the Council, 2002). A second programme was agreed (Decision of the European Parliament and of the Council, 2007) covering the period 2008–13, with three objectives: to improve citizens' health security, to promote health for prosperity and solidarity (including the reduction of health inequities), and to generate and disseminate health information and knowledge. These programmes of work were allocated funding (the second programme, for example, had a budget of €321 million). Examples of work funded by these programmes included the following: information exchange on health threats and preparedness plans; promoting health impact assessment of policies; healthy lifestyle campaigns; an overview of child obesity initiatives; the exchange of good practice on nutrition and physical activity; the development of good practice on alcohol and the workplace; support for HIV/AIDS networks and groups; support for initiatives to build capacity in the field of tobacco control; the prevention of illicit drug use; and the collection of data about health behaviours, diseases and conditions.

Box 2.2	**EU institutions and public health**

Several EU bodies are involved in public health governance. Within the European Commission (which proposes, develops and implements policy and legislation) there is a Directorate for Health and Consumers. Health issues also impinge on the work of other Directorates, such as Agriculture and Rural Development, Environment, Transport, Climate Action, Employment, Social Affairs and Inclusion, Competition, Enterprise and Industry. There is also a number of EU agencies that deal with health matters, including the Executive Agency for Health and Consumers, which implements EU programmes in this field. In addition, there are various specialist agencies with a role in protecting public health and safety, such as the European Agency for Safety and Health at Work, the European Food Safety Agency, the European Environment Agency, the Food and Veterinary Office, the European Chemicals Agency and the European Medicines Agency. Other important bodies include the European Centre for Disease Prevention and Control, which manages disease surveillance and responses, identifies emerging health threats, provides scientific advice, publishes research and provides training in this field. A specific body (the European Monitoring Centre for Drugs and Drug Addiction) exists to monitor drugs misuse.

The European Parliament also takes an interest in health and related matters and can raise issues and influence legislation. A specialist standing committee on the Environment, Public Health and Food Safety keeps these issues under scrutiny, examines legislative proposals, produces reports and makes recommendations. Health issues are also considered in other forums, such as the Committee of the Regions (an advisory body comprising representatives from Europe's regions, major cities and local authorities) and the Economic and Social Committee (which represents employers, trade unions, consumers and other interests).

The Council of Ministers (also known as the Council of the EU) can make important policy decisions on health issues. The Council, which is made up of ministers from member states, is configured differently depending on the issues under consideration. The Employment, Social Policy, Health and Consumer Affairs Council, which is the main decision-making body for health issues, involves ministers of health, social services, consumer affairs and employment. Other formations of the Council (such as Agriculture and Fisheries, and Environment) also make decisions that affect health. The Council of the EU is supported and coordinated by a body of officials drawn from each member state, known as COREPER (the Committee of Permanent Representatives). Council meetings are chaired and organized by the Presidency, which is held by a different member state every 6 months. Presidencies have identified health issues as priorities, and this has influenced the EU's agenda, especially in the past decade. The strategic direction of the EU is shaped by another body with a similar name, the European Council. The European Council consists of the heads of member states and now has its own elected President. Another key institution is the European Court of Justice, which interprets EU legislation. Its case law judgements across a range of issues (such as the environment, employment, competition, the regulation of products and services, and cross-border matters) can affect health in important ways. For example, European Court judgements on restrictions on the marketing of alcohol and tobacco have affected policies in all member states.

This might sound impressive. However, looked at another way, the funding allocated is small compared with the overall size of the EU budget (€123 billion in 2010). Moreover, most of the projects have been small and specific. One might well question how they could produce the significant shifts in policy needed to make public health a top priority for the EU. At the time of writing, a third programme covering the period 2014–20 has been proposed, with a budget of €446 million and four key objectives: to contribute to innovative and sustainable healthcare systems, to increase access to better and safer healthcare, to promote good health and prevent disease, and to protect citizens from cross-border health threats.

The increasing political visibility of health problems such as obesity, alcohol and smoking, coupled with a growing awareness of the links between health, economic efficiency and competitiveness (related to the EU's Lisbon agenda, linking social policy and competitiveness), and in the light of threats to the health of European citizens from beyond its borders, led the EU to consider a more strategic approach (Byrne, 2004). In 2007, the European Commission introduced a health strategy (Commission of the European Communities, 2007) that set out fundamental principles of EU action in health: shared health values, health as a prerequisite for economic activity, and the integration of health in all policies. A fourth principle, discussed further below, was to strengthen the voice of the EU in global health. The Commission also identified strategic aims, fostering good health in ageing populations, protecting citizens from health threats, and supporting health systems and new technologies. Proposed actions included: the adoption of a statement on fundamental health values, a system of health indicators, action on reducing health inequities, health literacy programmes, studies of the relationship between health and economic growth, strengthening the integration of health across EU policies, and strengthening cooperation between the EU and global health policy actors. The Council of Ministers (Box 2.2) agreed with the strategy and underlined its commitment with a declaration on 'health in all policies' at an EU Interministerial conference in Rome in 2007 (EU Ministerial Conference, 2007). The Council of Ministers also agreed that the EU should play a greater role in global public health (as noted above). This highlighted the need to take action to improve health, reduce inequality and increase protection against global health threats, to recognize health as a key element in sustainable growth and development and poverty reduction, and to call for 'increased leadership' of the WHO in global health.

Since the 2007 strategy, EU interest in health has grown further. To some extent, this has been due to the environmental health agenda, particularly issues relating to air pollution. There has also been much interest in tackling health inequalities and the social determinants of health. Both of these policy areas have created a stronger momentum towards 'health in all policies' and the promotion of intersectoral working on health. In addition, the Lisbon Treaty, which came into force in 2009, amended the EU's health responsibilities and powers in several ways. First, well-being was identified as a key aim of the EU. Second, the Treaty emphasized greater cooperation between member states to improve health services in cross-border areas. Third, it strengthened cooperation and coordination through guidelines, indicators, exchange of good practice, periodic monitoring and evaluation. Fourth, it confirmed that EU legislation would be permitted when setting high standards where there were common safety concerns (three areas were specified: blood products, organ transplants and other substances of human origin; medical products and devices; and measures in relation to animal or plant health with a direct objective of protecting public health). Fifth, EU competence in relation to cross-border health scourges and the protection of public health from alcohol and tobacco was clarified, allowing incentives to be used, but not legislation to harmonize laws.

Problems of governance and partnership

Despite the growing interest in health issues shown by EU institutions, and the greater priority given to this in EU legislation, documents and programmes, there are significant shortcomings in how health policy is developed and implemented. Although health is on the agenda of many EU bodies, it is not a top priority. The EU's role in health remains restricted by the Treaties (Greer, 2009a). Although many health-related provisions have been introduced, they have not until recently been part of any coherent strategy on health. A related problem is that EU health programmes have been underresourced. There has been, and to a large extent still is, a diffusion of governance on health (Lear and Mossialos, 2008), with a lack of clear authority and accountability for health actions. There is also poor coordination between the directorates and agencies whose activities impinge on health (Greer, 2009a). Although one can identify issues where great efforts have been made to promote a collaborative or partnership approach (such as drug abuse, where specific EU bodies have been established), this is relatively unusual.

Health came late to the EU agenda and has struggled to compete with established issues such as agriculture, industry, trade and competition, and even welfare and environment issues. Commercial interests are very powerful within the EU and skilled at opposing policies that might undermine their profitability. They have strong links with the most powerful economic and trade directorates within the European Commission. Drugs companies, agricultural interests and food, drink and alcohol corporations are particularly influential. Although there are examples of where the EU has developed policies that have offended some member states and business interests (for example, health warnings on tobacco products and restrictions on marketing), there are spectacular failures. Health issues have had no discernible impact on the Common Agricultural Policy, which has enormous implications for health through nutrition and diet (Elinder et al., 2003).

Nonetheless, public health groups have become more knowledgeable about EU activities and lobbying from these quarters has become more sophisticated. These interests have taken opportunities to interact with EU decision-makers. For example, there is a Health Policy Forum, established in 2001, which provides a vehicle for consultation on health issues. It consists of organizations representing trade unions, health professionals, health service providers and insurers, patients and consumers, and commercial interests. The forum identifies key areas of work within the context of an annual plan, examines specific issues and can adopt policy positions. In the light of criticism, however, new guiding principles on transparency were outlined for Health Policy Forum members (EU Health Policy Forum,

2007), including provisions on openness, conflicts of interest and governance. Subsequently, the Health Policy Forum was reformed in 2009. Its mandate was renewed with the following aims: that the membership should concentrate on pan-European rather than national or regional associations, that preference should be given to umbrella bodies able to represent a wider constituency of organizations, and that the membership should not exceed around 50 groups.

There are other consultative processes that are used by the European Commission to build collaboration and partnership with stakeholders. An Open Health Forum includes a wider range of organizations than the Health Policy Forum. In addition, the EU Platform for Action on Diet, Physical Activity and Health, formed in 2005, and the European Alcohol and Health Forum, launched in 2007, aim to promote consensus and dialogue between different interests in these particular policy areas. Although they have provided the foundation for joint commitments, their impact on policy has been quite limited (Celia et al., 2010; Evaluation Partnership, 2010). They have tended to focus on areas of consensus, such as information and communication about risks and lifestyles. Thornier issues, such as regulation, tend to be avoided. Notably, commercial interests view these bodies far more positively than non-profit organizations, an indication perhaps of their inadequacy in meeting public health objectives. In addition, some academic observers have commented that these processes are rather tokenistic and inhibit open discussion (Greer, 2009a).

There is clearly scope for greater cooperation and collaboration within the EU on public health, and in recent years efforts have been made to improve this. Health was included in EU integrated impact assessment guidelines in 2002, which are meant to be applied to all major EU policies. In addition, the European Commission funded a new guide to health impact assessment (International Health Impact Assessment Consortium, 2004) and funded studies of its application and use (Wismar et al., 2007). But although health has been acknowledged as an important aspect of EU social, environmental and economic policies, health impact assessment has not been fully utilized (Lock and McKee, 2005; Salay and Lincoln, 2008). Major policies and programmes, notably the Common Agricultural Policy, are still not subject to health impact assessment. There are, however, efforts to remedy this. For example, proposals to reform the Common Agricultural Policy make reference to health issues, such as diet and nutrition, although it is unclear at present exactly how these considerations will be factored in (Communication from the Commission, 2010).

Finally, efforts have been made to improve coordination and cooperation between member states on health matters. The Open Method of Coordination (OMC), introduced in 2000, enabled member states to come together to build consensus on issues where they retained a high degree of autonomy. The aim was to promote convergence. In 2004, OMC was extended to health matters. Under OMC, member states set out policy positions and plans, and share them, providing opportunities to learn from each other's experiences. This provides a basis for action, although there is little evidence that it has had much impact (Greer, 2009a). In 2008, OMC was revamped to raise its profile, sharpen its focus and improve communication, coordination and mutual learning.

EU institutions such as the Council of Ministers and the Commission have a more formal role in agreeing health goals and indicators, and monitoring arrangements. Key objectives have been set in three areas: access, quality and sustainability (including a focus on shorter waiting times), effective prevention and health promotion, and reducing health inequalities. In addition, further coordination mechanisms specific to health have been introduced. An interservice group on public health was created in the 1990s to coordinate activities between different parts of the European Commission. Specific subgroups were established to improve coordination on particular issues such as HIV/AIDS, global health and environmental health. Furthermore, in 2008, a Working Party on public health was established by the Council of the EU. It was to act as a forum to discuss major strategic issues, consider issues arising for health systems and public health from the application of the Lisbon Treaty, contribute to a strategic vision for health and ensure continuity in political and strategic debates, identify priorities, objectives and actions, contribute to the Council's strategic debates and decisions, carry out scanning and reviews of health-related activities, and suggest how to improve the 'health in all policies' approach. This working party is supported by the Commission and reports to COREPER (Box 2.2).

WHO Europe

The WHO Regional Office for Europe has been a key exponent of collaborative working and partnerships in health (Ziglio et al., 2005). Its membership is wider than that of the EU so is valuable in building consensus and introducing initiatives across the continent. The WHO European Region has pursued the goal of improving collaboration in health in a number of ways: first, by tailoring WHO strategies and initiatives, such as healthy public policy and promoting intersectoral working and partnership, to the European setting; and second, by working with other cross-national bodies such as the EU and the Council of Europe.

The WHO Europe has formulated broad strategies on health. Its regional Health for All strategy set specific aims and targets for the continent (WHO Regional Office for Europe, 1985, 1993c, 1999a). More recently, it developed Health 2020, a European policy framework for supporting action across government and society for health and well-being (WHO Regional Office for Europe, 2012b). In addition, it has developed a consensus enabling the formulation of specific resolutions, charters, strategies and action plans on a range of issues including alcohol, smoking, children's health, health systems, environmental health, non-communicable diseases, food and nutrition (WHO Regional Office for Europe, 1988, 1990, 1993a, 1993b, 1999b, 2000a, 2000b, 2001, 2004, 2006a, 2006b, 2010, 2011, 2012a). Other WHO Europe activities include programmes and projects such as Healthy Cities, Healthy School and Healthy Hospital initiatives, which seek to promote health through the involvement of these sectors. Furthermore, WHO Europe's Verona Initiative of the late 1990s was specifically geared to promoting collaboration in health across different sectors and inspired a number of projects in member states, including the UK.

Partnership and collaboration feature strongly in WHO Europe's work. For example, this is embedded in specific projects, such as Healthy Cities. Strategies and action plans relating to particular health problems and challenges also refer to collaboration and partnership. For example, the European Action Plan on the Prevention and Control of Non-communicable Diseases makes reference to the importance of these factors, notably intersectoral working and community empowerment. They also feature strongly in Health 2020, which refers to the importance of working across sectors, addressing social and environmental determinants of health, and increasing the participation of all stakeholders, including citizens, in improving health.

The Council of Europe

The Council of Europe is not an EU body (and is not to be confused with similarly named EU institutions, the European Council and the Council of the EU). It was founded in 1949 to uphold democracy, human rights and the rule of law and has 47 member states. Like WHO Europe, the fact that its membership includes non-EU states means that it is useful for getting agreement on issues across the European continent. The principal focus of the Council of Europe with regard to health is upon citizen's rights to health and healthcare and participation. For example, it has promoted action on issues such as nutrition, HIV/AIDS and elderly and disabled people. It has cooperated with other European institutions such as EU bodies and the WHO Regional Office for Europe on issues including school-based health promotion, drug dependence, hazardous chemicals, and the safety of blood products and organs for transplant.

Public health partnerships in other countries

In recent decades, public health issues have attracted greater interest across most countries. Many have devised strategies and/or have reformed their public health systems (Allin et al., 2004). Although these efforts have been diverse, there are some common themes, including intersectoral working, partnerships and collaboration. This section explores the experiences of several countries in establishing such arrangements, illustrating how other states are responding to similar challenges to those faced by the UK.

Canada

Canada is regarded as a pioneer in modern public health (Pederson et al., 2005). In the 1970s, a landmark report called for a greater recognition of the influence on health of factors outside the healthcare system (Lalonde, 1974). Canada was one the first countries to embrace key Health for All principles such as healthy public policy, intersectoral working, participation in health and equity in health. However, while recognizing the need to apply these principles, Canadian governments struggled to move beyond rhetoric and actually implement policies (Pederson et al., 2005; Raphael and Bryant, 2006). In Canada's system of government, responsibilities for public health are divided between the federal government, the provinces and territories, and local government. It proved diffi-cult to translate national objectives into provincial and local action, and the federal government was unable to exercise strong leadership (Allin et al., 2004). Notably, partnership has an additional dimension in Canada and in other federal systems: the 'partnership' between the different tiers of government is a crucial factor in achieving policy objectives.

Weaknesses in the public health system were exposed in the SARS outbreak in 2003, in which 44 people died in Canada. Consequently, there were calls (Canadian Institutes for Health Research, 2003; National Advisory Committee on SARS and Public Health, 2003; Senate Committee on Social Affairs, Science and Technology, 2003) for stronger leadership and greater coherence in public health governance, along with more resources, and it was acknowledged that a greater effort was needed to build collaboration between different agencies and organizations to enhance health protection and improvement. This led to the creation of a new federal public health agency in 2004 (the Public Health Agency of Canada), bringing together important areas of expertise on disease prevention and health promotion and led by a Chief Public Health Officer, accountable to the Minister of Health for Canada. The key objectives of the Public Health Agency of Canada are to provide leadership, promote partnership, stimulate innovation and drive forward action on public health. It has high-lighted the importance of collaboration between the different levels of govern-ment and between the various sectors that can influence health (see its website: www.phas-aspc.gc.ca). Furthermore, in 2005, a Pan-Canadian Public Health Network was created, bringing together government agencies, scientific experts and voluntary organizations to provide advice, information and support for those undertaking public health interventions (Ministry of Health Canada, 2005). A key role of the network is to prepare, implement and maintain inter-governmental arrangements on public health.

The federal government endorsed strategies on public health issues, such as cancer control, diabetes, heart health, HIV/AIDS, smoking and drug abuse, empha-sizing the importance of collaboration and partnership. These strategies emerged out of partnerships and coalitions of interest, encouraged by the federal govern-ment, between professional groups, government agencies and voluntary organiza-tions. Partnership and collaboration has also been a feature of broader health strategies. In 2005, the federal government launched an overarching strategy on healthy living and chronic disease (Minister of Health (Canada), 2005). This sought to promote health by addressing conditions that led to unhealthy lifestyles, to prevent chronic disease by focused and integrated action on disease and risk factors, and to extend early detection and monitoring of health and disease. Partnership working was identified as a key element in this programme, and an intersectoral healthy living network was funded as part of the federal government's package.

Partnership working has also been identified as a key issue at provincial level (see, for example, Ministry of Health Services, British Columbia, 2005). There is also much activity at local level, with some exemplary work on promoting the healthy public policy agenda in Montreal (Quebec), Chinook (Alberta), the Interior Region of British Columbia and parts of Ontario (Raphael and Bryant, 2006).

Australia

Australia, like Canada, is a federal state. The states, territories and localities are responsible for frontline public health functions in disease prevention and health promotion. The federal government is responsible for strategy, guidance and funding. As in Canada, there is much scope for promoting vertical collaboration between the different levels of government as well as horizontal collaboration between agencies (Allin et al., 2004). Like Canada, Australia endorsed key Health for All principles and similarly struggled to implement them (Nutbeam, 1999; Hearn et al., 2005; Lin, 2007). Familiar concerns about fragmentation, lack of coordination and lack of consistency in public health policy have also arisen. This is despite impressive achievements in some states, such as Victoria, where public health interventions on road safety and tobacco control were pioneered (see Powles and Gifford, 1993). Individual states have tended to pursue their own strategies on issues such as alcohol and drugs, diet and obesity. However, public health policy developments increasingly operate within a national context.

In 1985, a Better Health Commission was established to explore possible strategies for disease prevention and health promotion. Three years later, the federal government set out goals and targets to reduce preventable deaths (Health Targets and Implementation Committee, 1988). However, this was criticized for not placing sufficient emphasis on the wider causes of ill health, nor did it improve coordination and collaboration between different authorities (Nutbeam et al., 1993). A subsequent strategy (Commonwealth Departments of Human Services and Health, 1994) was also criticized for not sufficiently addressing the socioeconomic and environmental causes of ill health (Nutbeam, 1999).

By this time, however, the federal government had recognized the importance of developing effective partnerships. It established a review of partnership working, which set guidelines for successful collaboration (Harris et al., 1995). A National Public Health Partnership, created in 1996, developed a more consistent, coherent and comprehensive approach, its brief including the development of a national agenda for public health, coordination of strategies and improvements in communication between different levels of government. This body was superseded in 2006, when two new federal committees were created to take forward the collaborative agenda: the Australian Health Protection Committee (to coordinate action on disasters, environmental health threats and communicable disease) and the Australian Population Health Development Principal Committee (to coordinate national efforts to prevent disease and promote health). Both operate under the auspices of the Australian Health Ministers' Advisory Committee, which advises the Australian Health Ministers' Conference (comprising the health ministers of federal, state and territorial governments).

The federal government has developed specific strategies in areas such as tobacco control, drugs and nutrition and diet. It has also continued to strengthen the foundations for collaborative working. Building on an earlier agreement between states and territories on promoting health, a national partnership agreement on preventive health was agreed in 2008, setting out targets and responsibilities for federal and state/territorial agencies. A review of public health was also undertaken, which produced recommendations for a higher priority for issues such as obesity, alcohol misuse, smoking-related illness and health inequalities (Australian Government, 2009). Major recommendations included a national prevention agency to advise on national strategy, monitor and evaluate policies and programmes, establish a research framework, undertake surveillance of key heath problems, and facilitate collaborative approaches. A key emphasis of the review was on shared responsibility in public health, recommending strategic partnerships at all levels of government, and including industry, employers, business, NGOs, research institutions and communities. The report also highlighted the importance of community engagement in settings such as schools, workplaces and the community. The Australian Government (2010) has begun to implement these recommendations, including the establishment of a national preventive health agency to coordinate efforts to prevent chronic disease.

The USA

Following a report from the Surgeon General (US Surgeon General, 1979), the US federal government devised a health strategy setting out over 200 targets across 15 priority areas to be achieved by 1990 (USDHHS, 1980). The strategy was subsequently revised with the publication of Healthy People 2000 and Healthy People 2010 (USDHHS, 1991, 2000). Despite this, US public health policy has been criticized on several grounds (Institute of Medicine, 1988, 2002; Lightsey et al., 2005; Tilson and Berkowitz, 2006; Raphael, 2008): an overemphasis on individual lifestyles, coupled with a failure to address socioeconomic and environmental causes of ill health; poor implementation of policies; a lack of coordination between different agencies; underresourcing of public health functions; and a lack of capacity in the public health workforce. Subsequently, there have been attempts to strengthen leadership in public health, reinforce links between health and other policy areas, and promote greater collaboration between agencies and other stakeholders. Notably, Healthy People 2010 placed emphasis on the importance of collaboration between sectors. This was reiterated in the revised Healthy People 2020 strategy published in 2010, alongside a greater acknowledgement of the socioeconomic determinants of ill health (USDHHS, 2010).

The US Institute of Medicine (1988, 2002) earlier called for a more strategic approach, with greater emphasis on partnership and collaboration, that could mobilize agencies, businesses and communities to meet public health goals. The Centres for Disease Control and Prevention (CDCP), which bring together expertise and information on public health at federal government level, established programmes to stimulate collaborative work on public health issues. For example, in 2003, a programme called Steps to a HealthierUS led to a number of communities receiving funding for tackling particular health problems such as obesity, smoking and health inequalities. This subsequently developed into the CDCP Healthy Communities programme. These programmes sought to mobilize communities to promote health and build partnerships between different state organizations, as well as involving the private sector and community groups. Partnerships operate in a range of settings including schools, workplaces, healthcare organizations and the wider community. Examples of specific projects developed through these programmes include implementing healthy food options in Mexican restaurants (Salinas, California), raising nutrition standards of school lunches (New York) and improving employee health (Thurston County, Washington).

Individual states also began to reform their public health infrastructure, which involved the establishment of more effective strategies and collaborative arrangements. Furthermore, specific public health problems such as HIV/AIDs, tobacco control, injury prevention and drug abuse provided a focus for collaborative action, and in some states additional funding was provided to facilitate this. These various initiatives promoted collaborative working arrangements, such as coalitions and partnerships (Butterfoss, 2007).

However, foundations also played an important role. The Robert Wood Johnson Foundation and the W.K. Kellogg Foundation funded 'Turning Point' partnerships in the late 1990s to rethink public health delivery and develop collaborative models for more effective interventions. Turning Point partnerships were established in 21 states and 43 communities (including Oklahoma, California, Minnesota, New Hampshire and Oregon). These collaborative partnerships were expected to develop plans for public health improvement. Typically, they focused on addressing the main causes of ill health and preventing chronic disease. In California, for example, there was an explicit recognition of the challenge of chronic disease, an awareness of socioeconomic and racial inequalities as key determinants of ill health, and an acknowledgement that the root causes of these problems must be addressed. Here, a twin-track approach was pursued that involved the strengthening of communities through efforts to build cohesion and the coordination of activities to combat fragmentation. Specific problems were targeted using this approach, including obesity and poor diet.

One of the main shortcomings of the US public health system has been the unwillingness of federal government to prioritize public health policies and ensure implementation at state and local levels. Part of the problem lies in the US political system, in which state and local autonomy is highly valued. The neoliberal character of recent US governments (notably under Reagan and Bush Senior and Junior), institutionalized the bias against federal state intervention. More recently, under President Obama, there has been a move towards a stronger leadership role for the federal government in public health matters (notably related to Let's Move, a child obesity initiative, championed by the First Lady, Michelle Obama). The Obama administration established a National Prevention, Health Promotion and Public Health Council to lead and coordinate prevention activities, comprising senior government officials drawn from across federal government departments and agencies. Its task is to design a national prevention and health promotion strategy in conjunction with communities across the country. The strategy will take a community health approach to prevention and well-being. In addition, a new Prevention and Public Health Investment Fund has been established to expand and sustain the public health infrastructure for the next 10 years. Meanwhile, a new foundation, Partnership for a Healthier America, has been formed to channel additional resources into promoting healthy lifestyles.

Finland

Finland has been at the forefront of developments in public health for many years. It adopted the Health for All approach in its national plans in the late 1980s (Tervonen-Goncalves and Lehto, 2004; Hogstedt et al., 2008). Finland is seen as a strong exponent of public health policy, supporting the shift from treatment to prevention (WHO Regional Office for Europe, 2002). It has adopted a series of health strategies that target the main causes of ill health, including social determinants, and emphasize the importance of intersectoral working. The Health 2015 strategy (Ministry of Social Affairs and Health, 2001) sets out a range of objectives to be achieved by 2015, which include the reduction of inequalities, improving child health and well-being, reducing smoking, alcohol and drug use, and reducing accidental and violent death. The strategy is closely monitored, with periodic and comprehensive evaluation.

The Health 2015 strategy identifies a range of government and non-government actors that have a role in delivering its objectives. It also identifies a clear role for citizens in improving their health. The strategy is therefore based on an acknowledgement of an intersectoral and collaborative approach. In recent years, efforts have been made to strengthen partnership working and to integrate health concerns in all policies, partly in response to weakness identified through policy evaluation (WHO Regional Office for Europe, 2002). At a national level, arrangements to coordinate health-related activities between government departments, and to ensure that health is reflected in policy decisions across government, were strengthened (Stahl et al., 2006). An advisory board of public health was created in the late 1990s to monitor and coordinate policy. Its members are drawn from government agencies, municipalities and non-government bodies. One of its three divisions deals specifically with intersectoral cooperation. In addition to this, ministries formally exchange information about the health-related activities, and these are supplemented with bilateral discussions to produce national public health reports. There is also a policy programme for health promotion, initiated in 2007, which is accountable to the prime minister's office. This seeks to promote intersectoral working at the municipal level, which had previously been identified as a weakness, given the autonomy of these bodies (WHO Regional Office for Europe, 2002). In addition, changes to made to public health legislation in 2006 placed requirements on local bodies to undertake intersectoral action (Hogstedt et al., 2008).

Cuba

In Cuba, health has been a national priority since the 1959 revolution (Kirk and Erisman, 2009), and health is seen as a human right. Cuban health outcomes – in terms of indicators such as life expectancy and infant mortality – are comparable to those found in Western industrialized nations (Feinsilver, 1993; Macintyre and Hadad, 2002). One of the reasons for its high performance in health relative to its level of economic development is that it has a universal healthcare system that is accessible and free (save some small out-of-pocket payments for medicines) to all its population (De Vos, 2005). Another is its strong primary care network, with highly localized family doctor services centred round polyclinics (Reed, 2008). Third, there is a strong emphasis on public health and the need to prevent illness by addressing social, economic and environmental determinants of health (Evans, 2008).

The Cuban system places great weight on collaboration and partnership. In 1989, a healthy municipalities strategy was launched to tackle social determinants of health, involve communities and improve planning across sectors (Spiegel and Yassi, 2004). Health Councils were formed in 1995 to integrate different sectors (Feinsilver, 2010). These appear to have strengthened collaboration between agencies in different sectors (Spiegel et al., 2012). In addition, integration is enhanced by municipal and provincial directors of public health serving as vice presidents of their respective levels of government administration (Castell-Florit, 2010).

Another key aspect of the Cuban system is its emphasis on public participation (Feinsilver, 1993; Kath, 2011). This takes a number of forms. Mass organizations (such as the Committees for the Defense of the Revolution, trade unions and women's organizations) raise health issues. In addition, there are local citizen action groups that focus on health matters. Elected bodies (Poder Popular) consider health issues, and people can discuss matters with delegates. Neighbourhood committees can also raise issues and participate in health needs analysis and planning. It should be noted that participation in the Cuban health system is a two-way process. While there are opportunities for citizens to raise issues, there are also mechanisms for mobilizing the community (Greene, 2003). Indeed, some argue that this is really the primary purpose of popular participation (Feinsilver, 2010; Kath, 2011). Nonetheless, such mobilization forms an important part of health campaigns, including health promotion activities and measures to prevent infectious disease.

The Cuban health system is embedded in a very different political system from the other countries mentioned in this section and is at a different level of income and economic development. There are also political barriers to learning from its example, and practical issues around undertaking and validating research into the benefits (and also the costs) of the Cuban system. Nonetheless, it offers a number of lessons and suggestions for how intersectoral working, collaboration and partnership could be improved.

Conclusion

This chapter has shown that issues of public health leadership, partnership and collaboration are extremely important at the global and international level. It is acknowledged that more must be done, not only to prioritize public health issues at this level, but also to develop and implement coherent strategies and programmes. Moreover, the search is on for more effective and accountable ways of delivering public health objectives through partnership and collaboration. Compared with models of collaborative and partnership working, outlined in Chapter 1, global and international efforts fall considerably short, particularly on the degree to which policies are evaluated for their health impact and the influence of health and well-being objectives in non-health policy sectors. However, at present there are stronger pressures to strengthen processes and institutions, at global and at European level.

Individual countries have also acknowledged that public health objectives merit higher priority. They have recognized the difficulties of partnership and collaborative working and have devised different ways of overcoming them. There is much variation between countries, even at a similar level of economic development. Some of these differences derive from different political cultures and systems. However, there are also strong similarities among these states in their efforts to strengthen and develop partnership working and intersectoral collaboration. Their experience illustrates the scale of the challenge to ensure that health and well-being considerations are given due weight within a collaborative and intersectoral process. There are also positive lessons. Some countries have achieved gains by setting clear objectives and priorities, demonstrating leadership and promoting intersectoral working through partnership and engagement processes. There is thus considerable scope for lesson-drawing here, which has so far not been fully exploited.

3 Partnerships under New Labour

Introduction

As noted in Chapter 1, the New Labour governments placed great emphasis on partnership working, with the aim of promoting 'joined-up government'. However, partnerships tended to evolve rather than being shaped by a clear blueprint. Indeed, with regard to partnerships on health and well-being, the policy was essentially an accumulation of several policy streams. First, central government policies on public health, including White Papers and related structural and procedural changes, identified coordination and partnership as a means of achieving objectives in this field. Second, specific public health problems were identified as needing a collaborative approach. Third, health programmes and schemes were introduced that included partnership as a key element. Fourth, policies on the relationship between the NHS and social care had important implications for other partnerships. Fifth, a range of wider policies in the NHS and local government, as well as specific programmes and performance management processes, promoted partnership working. Sixth, policies emerging in other policy sectors encouraged partnership working with health bodies. This chapter explores these various factors and how they shaped the development of partnerships in health and well-being. It also explores the impact of these policies on partnership working in practice. The primary focus is on policy developments in England. However, towards the end of the chapter, specific policies relating to Scotland, Wales and Northern Ireland are discussed.

Central government and public health policy

In opposition, Labour argued that public health policy lacked priority and was poorly coordinated. On taking office, it introduced changes at national level, including a minister for public health and a new Cabinet committee to improve coordination. In 1999, a new public health White Paper was published, *Saving Lives: Our Healthier Nation* (Cm 4386, 1999), which identified new targets for reducing major causes of illness and death, to be achieved by 2010:

■ To reduce the death rate from heart disease, stroke and related illnesses among people aged under 75 years by at least two-fifths.
■ To reduce the death rate from accidents by at least a fifth and reduce the rate of serious injury by at least a tenth.
■ To reduce the death rate from cancer among people aged under 75 by at least a fifth.
■ To reduce the death rate from suicide and undetermined injury by at least a fifth.

Compared with the previous government's strategy, New Labour's plans gave greater attention to socioeconomic and environmental factors (although John Major's government did announce a plan to add the environment to its *Health of the Nation* strategy shortly before the 1997 General Election). New Labour also explicitly identified the need to build strong partnerships between the state and individuals, central government and local agencies, the NHS and other local bodies, stating that:

> The goals of this health strategy will be achieved only by a joint effort. That means individuals taking steps to improve their own health, and on new directions and new more effective partnerships formed at local community level between the NHS, local authorities and other agencies. (Cm 4386, 1999, p. 119)

Saving Lives mentioned specific programmes that would make such partnerships a reality. These included Health Action Zones (HAZs) and Healthy Living Centres (HLCs), discussed below. The White Paper also made it clear that NHS bodies and planning processes would give higher priority to public health issues and to working in partnership with others.

The impact of *Saving Lives* was minimal, however. In reality, public health did not become a higher priority. Partnership working remained variable across the country. Subsequently, a further White Paper, *Choosing Health*, was produced (Cm 6374, 2004). This focused more on risk factors associated with the major causes of illness and death (such as smoking, alcohol misuse and obesity), harking back to the Conservatives' White Paper *The Health of the Nation*. The key theme of *Choosing Health* was to support individuals in making healthy choices about their lifestyles. Coordination between different agencies was again identified as crucial to the achievement of public health objectives. This White Paper envisaged a key role for networks of local health champions, drawn from the NHS, local government and the voluntary and private sectors. It identified a role for the private sector in helping people make healthier choices, for example in terms of diet, drinking and exercise (see Chapter 7). New schemes to promote collaborative working were launched, discussed further below. Another theme of *Choosing Health* was to develop the capacity of the public health workforce and strengthen the contribution of professional groups across different agencies to public health (discussed further in Chapter 4).

Choosing Health promised that a Cabinet committee on public health, first established under John Major, would be revitalized and that health would become more fully integrated in decision-making across government. In a further attempt to re-establish public health as a priority and strengthen cross-departmental working, the government upgraded the minister of public health post (previously downgraded in ministerial rank when its first incumbent moved to another post).

Specific public health issues

Much impetus for coordination and partnership came as a response to specific public health issues. Arguing that the previous government had failed to coord-inate policy on food and health, perhaps most notably on the issue of 'mad cow disease' (bovine spongiform encephalopathy in cattle and its link with Creutzfeldt–Jakob disease in humans), Labour decided to create an independent food agency. The Food Standards Agency was duly established in 2000 to develop, coordinate and implement policy on food safety and nutrition. Other agencies were also established to improve coordination on key public health issues – such as the Health Protection Agency, formed in 2003 from several agencies involved in preventing and responding to outbreaks of communicable diseases and biological, radiation and chemical hazards.

As it became clear that national policies alone would not bring the scale of improvement that government had envisaged, further attempts were made to improve the coordination of policy and partnership arrangements at local level. For example, with regard to smoking cessation, government promoted local alli-ances to bring together existing organizations. With regard to obesity also, it became obvious that local bodies (such as schools, councils, NHS bodies and the private and voluntary sectors) must work more closely together. Alcohol was another issue that merited closer working between local agencies such as the police, the probation service, NHS, local authorities, employers, alcohol agencies and other voluntary organizations (see Thom et al., 2013).

To support such activities, local public health networks were established to build capacity and secure economies of scale in public health. They were intended as a means of overcoming problems of fragmentation by building collaboration (Evans, 2003; Hunter et al., 2007). They also supported professional development in public health. Networks can operate in a single local area or across a wider region (see LGA and DH, 2012). Members are mainly drawn from NHS bodies and include health-care professionals and managers, as well as academics, voluntary organizations and local authorities. Although informal, these networks have had an impact on building collaboration on issues such as professional development, and tackling specific public health issues such as smoking, obesity and alcohol problems. Some have been very successful in influencing commissioning, promoting information- and data-sharing, and pooling skills and resources. In some cases, they have provided a platform for developing and delivering public health programmes. However, their coverage has been patchy, there has been a lack of consensus over their main purpose, they have not been well resourced, and they have been given a low priority (Abbott et al., 2005; Connelly et al., 2005; Fotaki, 2007).

Public health partnership programmes

In 1998, a programme of HAZs was launched to improve interagency collaboration on health in areas of high need (Powell and Moon, 2001; Matka et al., 2002; Barnes et al., 2005; Judge and Bauld, 2007). A total of 26 HAZs were created, covering 13 million people. They aimed to address public health needs, improve efficiency, effectiveness and responsiveness, develop partnerships for health improvement and service provision, integrate services, reduce health inequalities and engage with local communities. Schemes varied enormously. Some focused on improving relationships between healthcare and social care services; others were more geared to health promotion objectives such as smoking cessation. The aims of the HAZs were ambitious, and they operated in a relatively short time frame with limited resources. In 2003, they were absorbed into Primary Care Trusts (PCTs).

HLCs were introduced in 1998 to improve health and well-being in deprived communities. Based on partnerships between NHS bodies, local government and voluntary organizations, and receiving funding from the National Lottery, these projects aimed to integrate health and social welfare services, including childcare, counselling, employment advice, youth services and health promotion. Not all projects were, however, based in a single centre or building. Some constituted networks bringing together a range of agencies and functions. Over 300 HLCs were funded over a five-year period. The expectation was that funding would be continued by local agencies, but this did not always happen and some facilities were reduced or even closed down.

A number of other programmes had partnership building as a key aim. For example, the Healthy Communities collaborative, launched in 2000, focused initially on multiagency efforts to prevent falls in elderly people and later applied to other issues, such as improving diets among disadvantaged groups. The Communities for Health programme, which began in 2004, consisted of locally authority-led partnership initiatives on issues such as obesity, sexual health, cancer, alcohol misuse and smoking (see also Box 5.4). Starting in 2006, the Healthy Communities programme aimed to build local authority capacity and leadership on public health and promote joined-up working. In addition, guidance on partnerships was produced by central government (ODPM and DH, 2005). National support teams for joint PCT/local authority initiatives were also established. In 2008, a further programme, Healthy Towns, was introduced. This introduced two-year pilot projects to promote partnership working across local agencies to improve diet, increase physical activity and reduce obesity. Examples included a project in Manchester that rewarded people for undertaking physical activity, and another in Halifax that encouraged citizens to grow their own fruit and vegetables. Labour also introduced Healthy Places, Healthy Lives in 2009 to develop a joint approach between local public services in 30 sites to address the social determinants of health and reduce inequalities.

NHS, local authorities and social care reforms

Policies on public health partnerships were shaped by wider reforms in health and social care. The Blair government recognized that relationships between the NHS and social care providers had often been poor (see Wistow, 2012, and Chapter 1). In the 1999 Health Act, a revised statutory duty of cooperation was imposed on NHS bodies and local councils. This built on an existing duty (introduced by the NHS Reorganisation Act of 1973) that, in exercising their functions, health authorities and local authorities 'shall cooperate with one another in order to secure and advance the health and welfare of the people of England and Wales'. Cooperation was not, however, confined to social care matters (which had traditionally dominated the health–social care interface) but included public health. National guidance on partnership working (DH, 1998b) and on joint health and social care priorities (DH, 1998c) allocated lead responsibilities on specific health and social care matters. NHS bodies were required to involve local authorities and voluntary organizations in planning, including new local health plans (initially known as Health Improvement Programmes, later renamed Health Improvement and Modernization Plans). Local authorities were given a statutory duty to participate in the formulation and review of these plans and were expected to have regard to these plans. At the same time, the previous system of Joint Consultative Committees and joint finance (see Chapter 1) was abolished. In addition, different local agencies came together to draw up joint investment plans for those who used a range of NHS, local and voluntary sector services (such as elderly people and people with mental illness). The role of non-NHS organizations was further recognized in the development of National Service Frameworks, which outlined service standards and goals for particular conditions (such as coronary heart disease and mental illness) and groups of users (including children and elderly people). National Service Frameworks covered prevention and social care, as well as healthcare services, and sought to promote an integrated response to both health and social care needs.

Structures, processes and performance management

Partnership working also began to feature in performance and management systems in both NHS and local government. Within the NHS, this was formalized by the inclusion of partnership working in the Standards for Better Health (DH, 2006a). These standards explicitly included an expectation that healthcare would be provided in partnership with other organizations. Moreover, in the context of a new statutory duty on NHS bodies (in the 2001 Health and Social Care Act) to secure the involvement and consultation of the public and service users, the standards stated that healthcare must be provided in partnership with patients, carers and relatives (explored further in Chapter 5). With regard to public health and the reduction of health inequalities, the standards stated that healthcare organizations must cooperate with each other and with local authorities and other organizations, and make appropriate contributions to local partnership arrangements. The nature of these arrangements is discussed later in this chapter.

In the 1999 Health Act, the Blair government sought to create stronger financial incentives to encourage partnership in health and social care, giving NHS and local government bodies more flexibility to pool budgets, transfer funds and delegate functions to each other. In addition, it created new care trusts to arrange and provide both health and social care services for particular groups (such as older people, people with mental illness and people with learning disabilities; Glasby and Peck, 2003). Only a small number of these organizations were, however, created, partly because of the hostility from existing organizations, particularly local authorities, and practical barriers to their establishment (such as difficulties in transferring functions and staff to the NHS from local government).

Other structural changes were relevant to the partnership agenda. After taking office in 1997, the Labour government established Primary Care Groups to take on the role of commissioning healthcare. It was hoped that, by including local authority representatives on these bodies, partnership working would improve. The government expected that Primary Care Groups would gradually evolve into PCTs – larger, statutory bodies with more powers and responsibilities that included the provision of primary care. Nonetheless, PCTs were imposed in all areas by 2002 and given substantial responsibilities for the NHS budget. As they developed, PCTs were expected to work more closely with other local agencies. Their widespread creation coincided with the abolition of health authorities. Consequently, PCTs acquired additional public health powers, making them vital to the development of local public health policy, planning, coordination and service delivery. For example, they were expected to devise local health plans, undertake statutory public health functions, participate in local partnership forums and pilot new policies on public health, especially in deprived areas. PCTs were also responsible for appointing and employing local Directors of Public Health (DPHs) and their teams (with appointments of DPHs increasingly involving local authorities in the process).

The importance of partnership working was reiterated in the latter years of New Labour's time in office. A further White Paper, *Our Health, Our Care, Our Say* (Cm 6737, 2006), underlined the importance of PCTs in promoting health and preventing illness, and the need for local agencies to work together, as well as with service users and the public. It endorsed joint NHS–local authority appointments and multiagency teams, and supported moves to jointly assess needs and undertake commissioning of services on this basis. This led to the introduction of a new statutory joint assessment process of health and well-being – the Joint Strategic Needs Assessment (JSNA). This, along with developments in Local Area Agreements (LAAs; see below), led to new structures of collaboration on health (DH, 2007a). Many local areas formed health and well-being partnership boards, including representatives from local public sector bodies and the private and voluntary sectors. Councils, NHS bodies and their partners also began to develop local health strategies, covering issues such as smoking, obesity and alcohol, with partnership arrangements to secure key priorities.

The importance of joint needs assessment and commissioning was reiterated by the Darzi Review (Cm 7432, 2008). Darzi called for closer working between NHS and local government to promote and maintain health, as well as provide a more integrated system of health and social care. He also recommended greater investment in health promotion and comprehensive health and well-being services. Finally, developments in health service commissioning had implications for partnership working, with the advent of World Class Commissioning (DH, 2007b). This programme aimed to raise standards of commissioning across several areas of capacity, skill and competence. Several of these were highly relevant to public health and partnership working – notably leadership, prioritizing investment, knowledge management and needs assessment, collaborative working and public engagement.

Box 3.1	Joined-up action on health inequalities

In 2001, the Blair government undertook a cross-cutting review of health inequalities, in the light of its decision to set targets in this field. A cross-departmental action plan was produced (DH, 2003) that set out actions in four areas: supporting families, mothers and children; engaging communities and individuals; preventing illness and providing effective treatment and care; and addressing the underlying determinants of health and the long-term causes of health inequalities. Key outcome targets for health inequalities were set: to reduce by at least 10 per cent the gap in infant mortality deaths between 'routine and manual' groups and the population as a whole; and to reduce by at least 10 per cent the gap in life expectancy at birth between the fifth of local areas with the worst health and deprivation and the population as a whole. A number of other targets and indicators relating to health inequalities were also set (for example, reducing inequalities in certain diseases and risk factors, such as cardiovascular disease and smoking). In addition, the importance of reducing health inequalities was mentioned in strategic planning documents (such as the NHS planning framework) and additional resources were provided for health initiatives in deprived areas. Action on health inequalities was also integral to programmes such as Communities for Health and Healthy Places, Healthy Lives (see main text).

Despite efforts to prioritize health inequalities and encourage intersectoral efforts to reduce them, the outcome was disappointing. In the case of the life expectancy target, health inequalities actually widened (by 7 per cent in men and 17 per cent in women; DH, 2011a). The gap in infant mortality rates also widened initially but then narrowed (DH, 2010a), enabling this target to be met by 2010 (DH, 2010a, 2011f). The government was criticized for not doing enough to reduce health inequalities (see, for example, Healthcare Commission and Audit Commission, 2008; Health Committee, 2009; Audit Commission, 2010a; PAC, 2010). It was argued that there were too many short-term initiatives, shifts in policy, and unclear policy objectives as well as poor evaluation. It was found that, in reality, health inequalities lacked priority within performance management frameworks and that insufficient resources were allocated. Furthermore, not enough was done to address underlying social and economic inequalities and the social determinants of health. Intersectoral collaboration and partnership working were also identified as areas of weakness (see also Exworthy and Hunter, 2012). Although there had been some improvements in local partnership working in this field, they were not on the scale needed to address the issue. One problem was poor integration between policies that sought to reduce inequalities with those that aimed to improve healthy lifestyles. Indeed, a study by the King's Fund (Buck and Frosini, 2012) found that although the proportion of the population engaging in three or four unhealthy behaviours (smoking, excessive alcohol use, poor diet and low levels of physical activity) had fallen from a third to a quarter between 2003 and 2008, the gap between higher socioeconomic and educational groups and those in lower social groups had actually widened.

Partnership working with other sectors

Although much momentum for improvements in partnership working came from developments within health policy, other policy arenas were also influential. Policies aimed at reducing poverty and disadvantage contained a strong element of partnership and collaboration. These included policies on regeneration and neighbourhood renewal, such as New Deal for Communities and the Neighbourhood Renewal Strategy, as well as those addressing poverty and inequality. Although the Labour government was criticized for not doing enough to reduce deprivation, poverty and inequality, it at least created a framework that acknowledged the multidimensional and intersectoral nature of these and other intractable problems. Central institutions and processes were established to promote a more collaborative approach on a range of cross-departmental issues (Parker et al., 2010). The government initiated cross-sector reviews and set out targets and action plans across departments, for example on health inequalities (Box 3.1). In addition, delivery systems increasingly emphasized collaborative working and partnerships. Public Service Agreements between the Treasury and other government departments included issues that spanned traditional departmental boundaries (such as child obesity) and set targets and priorities that hitherto tended to be ignored as a result of the dominant 'silo mentality'. In some cases, national policy units were established to guide and support the implementation of policy (for example, on teenage pregnancy). Government-wide policies on specific client groups were also influential in promoting a more joined-up approach. Policies on child health and well-being (and child welfare more generally) provided a particularly important stimulus (Box 3.2).

The crime and policing agenda was another important driver of public health partnerships. Government sought to place greater emphasis on prevention of crime while trying to encourage a more community-oriented and interagency approach. This led to the creation of Crime and Disorder Reduction Partnerships (which became more commonly known as Community Safety Partnerships) at local level. These bodies, which incorporate a range of local agencies, have often become involved in public health issues. For example, road safety has been an important area of activity, with the introduction of interventions such as speed cameras and local speed limits. Alcohol- and drug-related problems have fallen within the remit of Community Safety Partnerships (and also Drug Action Teams, established to improve the coordination of drug, and increasingly alcohol, prevention and treatment services at local level). The increasing perception of binge drinking and its relationship to crime and disorder led many partnerships to promote interagency collaboration on issues such as alcohol licensing restrictions and enforcement, underage drinking, improvements in the drinking environment to minimize risk, the production of 'safer drinking' education materials and the referral of problem drinkers to counselling and support services. Illicit drugs have also been a focus of concern for partnership bodies, given the multidimensional nature of drug misuse problems, including crime, vice and ill health.

The expanding role of local government in health

One of the major developments after 1997 was the expansion of local government's role in health. This is particularly true of higher tier authorities (county councils), unitary authorities and London boroughs, which have social services responsibilities. However, district councils have an important public health function too, given their existing responsibilities for environmental health, housing, road safety and waste management, as well as other areas of regulation and service provision. The above-mentioned decision to reinforce local authority duties to cooperate with the NHS on matters of health and welfare, alongside flexibilities for pooled and delegated budgets, was important in drawing local government more closely into the health arena. In 2000, a further statutory duty was introduced on local authorities to draw up a community strategy that could include health issues. This was later subsumed into a duty to formulate a sustainable community strategy incorporating the 'green' agenda. Meanwhile, councils were granted new powers to promote or improve the economic, social and environmental well-being of their communities.

In addition, health scrutiny was introduced in 2003 (Coleman and Glendinning, 2004; NPCRDC, 2006). Councils providing social services were required to establish Health Overview and Scrutiny Committees (HOSCs) to scrutinize the planning, provision and operation of health services. HOSCs included council members and were allowed to co-opt others for specific inquiries. They were given two main functions. The first was to be consulted by the NHS on proposals to substantially change services (and if dissatisfied, HOSCs could refer such matters to the Secretary of State for Health). The second was to undertake reviews of health and healthcare issues. HOSCs were given powers to request information and require the attendance of NHS managers to give evidence.

Although seen as a welcome addition to the existing scrutiny function of local government, the effectiveness of HOSCs was questioned. In particular, it was believed that weaknesses found in other areas of local authority scrutiny – such as lack of resources, limited powers, lack of specialist knowledge and the conflict between councillors' roles (as public representative and party member) – would manifest themselves in relation to HOSCs. Research on HOSCs identified several similar shortcomings (Johnson et al., 2007; Boyd and Coleman, 2011), including lack of relevant technical knowledge in health, limited powers and insufficient support and resources for their role. In some situations, it was found that party politics rather than the public interest did come to the fore. This research also found that HOSCs had only a slight influence in changing NHS plans and services. However, it also found that influence should not be seen as a one-way/one-off process, and that HOSCs may have played a more subtle role in opening health services to scrutiny and external views. Notably, the influence of HOSCs varied across different issues. The style of scrutiny also varied, with more 'cooperative' approaches being more commonly found (and appropriate) to reviews of issues and policy, while 'adversary' approaches were more evident when service reorganizations were being considered. Although the principal focus of HOSCs has been on healthcare services, many have taken an opportunity to explore the public health agenda, including obesity, alcohol abuse, teenage pregnancy and health inequalities. In some cases, such inquiries raised the profile of these issues on council agendas. Indeed, some observers detected a shift from a narrow focus on specific services towards cross-cutting issues, including public health issues and matters affecting both health and social care (Johnson et al., 2007); and in the light of this experience, some councils merged their health scrutiny committees with those that scrutinized social care.

Further flexibility in scrutiny arrangements was promised by Cameron's Coalition government, which succeeded New Labour. As part of its emphasis on localism, it initially proposed that new Health and Wellbeing Boards (see Chapter 4) should undertake a health scrutiny role. This was dropped following concerns about the need to separate council executive and scrutiny functions. Instead, it was proposed that councils should retain the responsibility to organize scrutiny in ways best suited to their circumstances. Councils could retain HOSCs if they wished but would not be obliged to undertake health scrutiny through an overview and scrutiny committee. Moreover, it was proposed that the task of referring substantial changes in NHS services to the Secretary of State for Health be transferred from HOSCs to the full council (or to joint committees with other councils designated for that purpose). At the same time, councils' scrutiny powers were to be extended to all NHS-funded services (including independent providers of primary, community and hospital care).

Another factor leading to increased interest in the health agenda among councils was the initiation of changes to local partnership structures and processes. This reflected the role of local authorities as community leaders and 'place shapers' (Cm 6939, 2006). Rather than simply focusing on the services for which they were responsible, councils were expected to work with a range of agencies (including the private and voluntary sectors) to achieve national and local priorities. In order to provide an overarching framework for these partnerships, Local Strategic Partnerships (LSPs) were established in 2001, initially in areas receiving Neighbourhood Renewal funding. Although non-statutory, they were subsequently extended to all areas. While the membership of LSPs, and their governance arrangements, varied, they tended to include representatives from the main public bodies locally (for example, councils, the NHS, police and universities), as well as voluntary and private sectors. LSPs took on the role of producing the local sustainable community plan, seeking to ensure that all the local stakeholders agreed with and helped to implement it. In addition, they were responsible for developing LAAs. LAAs, introduced in 2004 initially on a pilot basis and from 2007 mandatory throughout England for all county councils, London boroughs and single-tier local authorities, were intended as a means of aligning the separate plans of various local bodies by specifying priorities, actions, resources and expected outcomes for the forthcoming three-year period. LSPs played an important part in producing consensus between local partners, and negotiating with the relevant Government Office for the Region (GOR; see below) for their area. In 2007, LSPs were strengthened by new obligations placed on local bodies to participate in the formulation and implementation of LAAs.

A further development was Comprehensive Area Assessment (CAA), introduced in 2009. The aim of CAA was to measure the performance of local public services in a holistic way, bringing together separate assessments of each service, involving a stronger focus on outcomes and identifying scope for improvement. The shift towards an area-based approach was continued by a further initiative, Total Place, introduced as a pilot scheme in 2009, which enabled local areas to set up projects exploring more efficient and effective ways of addressing priorities and specific problems by bringing together organizations and funding streams. Another initiative was participatory budgets, in which local residents and communities were given a say in decisions on budgets brought together from different sources.

Under Labour, local partnership working developed under strong pressure from central government. The various reforms already mentioned – LAAs, CAAs and LSPs – were centrally mandated. Central government established a stronger regional presence. GORs, established in the 1990s to join up the work of central government departments, became a stronger conduit of central policies. They had an important role in agreeing LAAs, for example, and in monitoring the performance of local authorities and the wider public sector in relation to targets and outcomes. Closer working arrangements between regional health bodies and regional government also developed. In 2002, regional directors of public health and their teams were relocated to GORs. In 2006, a reorganization of the NHS led to a reduction in the number of Strategic Health Authorities (SHAs), and as a result most had co-terminous boundaries with a single government regional office. This was widely regarded as strengthening the basis for coordination across the health and other policy areas. In addition, SHA directors of public health and regional director posts were combined, further strengthening the scope for joint working. Furthermore, guidance was issued to both GORs and SHAs to establish arrangements for improving health and well-being in their regions. Added to this, Labour had earlier established regional public health observatories to provide intelligence on public health and thereby facilitate and support multiagency initiatives to tackle health problems such as smoking, alcohol misuse, obesity and health inequalities.

The health role of local authorities has been strengthened further since these changes. The case for councils to lead and coordinate partnership working on issues such as health inequalities, tackling the social determinants of health, addressing environmental health factors and meeting the health challenges of modern urban settings has, if anything, become stronger (see Rydin, 2012; WHO Regional Office for Europe, 2012a). Moreover, as we shall see in the next chapter, significant new responsibilities for public health and well-being have been given to local authorities in England.

The impact of New Labour reforms on partnership working

It is difficult to assess the impact of New Labour's reforms on partnership working in public health. The reforms did not occur in a vacuum: other influences and policies were at work that might have had an impact (Hunter et al., 2011). Another problem is that policies and interventions were not comprehensively evaluated, a common complaint in both multiagency working generally and public health in particular (Wanless, 2004; Health Committee, 2009). Most important of all, there was little effort to evaluate outcomes (Smith, K. et al., 2009; Perkins et al., 2010; Hunter et al., 2011).

Nonetheless, some progress in partnership working between the NHS and local government on public health appears to have occurred from the late 1990s (NPCRDC, 2006; Audit Commission, 2007a; Healthcare Commission and Audit Commission, 2008). However, the quality of joint working varied considerably between local areas, and there was considerable scope for improvement (Audit Commission, 2007a, 2009; Wanless, 2007; Local Government Information Unit, 2010; Oneplace, 2010; Hunter et al., 2011). With regard to outcomes, a systematic review found no clear evidence that partnerships improved health, reduced disease or narrowed health inequalities. (Hunter et al., 2011).

Many of the generic factors enhancing partnership working (see Chapter 1) seem to be important in public health partnerships (Audit Commission, 2007a; Perkins et al., 2010; Hunter et al., 2011), for example, clear aims and strategy, a good history of collaboration between local agencies, trust and goodwill, clear account-abilities, awareness of roles and responsibilities, co-terminous boundaries, priorities and strategies, adequate resources, leadership, local health champions, involvement of senior management from key agencies, and a willingness to share information. In addition, the growing interest of local government in health may have been a posi-tive factor. The creation of HOSCs, for example, has been linked with improve-ments in partnership working on health (Local Government Information Unit, 2010), although there has been no systematic study of this effect. LSPs and LAAs have been regarded as important mechanisms for strengthening partnership working in public health (Healthcare Commission and Audit Commission, 2008). In 2009, the top 10 indicators selected for inclusion in LAAs included three health-related targets (Audit Commission, 2010a). However, according to Hunter et al. (2011), structures may be less important than underlying relational factors such as trust and goodwill. Moreover, concerns were expressed about the shortcomings of LAAs with regard to accountability, delivery, monitoring and measurement of progress towards targets (Hunter et al., 2011). LAA targets, CAA and place-based initiatives (such as Total Place and participatory budgets) heralded a more integrated approach across different agencies (Audit Commission, 2007a; Healthcare Commission and Audit Commission, 2008). However, it appears that individual organizations mostly continued to function as separate bodies with their own priorities and targets (Hunter et al., 2011). Findings from a review of CAA found that although many areas had given priority to improving health and some had been innovative, only a few had addressed the multiple challenges of economic regeneration, environ-mental sustainability and persistent inequalities (Oneplace, 2010).

Notably, some of these findings were reflected in the long-term evaluation of LAAs and LSPs (DCLG, 2011a), which revealed that LSPs were valuable arenas for sharing concerns, establishing a local collective vision and coordinating strategy. They could stimulate innovation in partnership working and provide a basis for service improvement and improved efficiency. Improvements in data-sharing were found, along with improved communication and a more coherent local voice. But there was less success in overcoming duplication and in pooling budgets. However, much depended on the nature and strength of trust and relationships. Leadership was also important in ensuring that partner organizations kept to their commitments. There was variation in the quality of partnerships. Cultural barriers remained and, along with limited resources and a lack of time, could impede partnership working. The disruptive impact of reorganizations on partnership working was also noted. A further issue was a lack of clarity about the accountability of LSPs and some uncertainty about where responsibility for delivery lay. LAAs were credited with moving away from a less silo-based towards a more joined-up approach to performance management. But there were problems with the quality of data, and although it was acknowledged that LAAs brought more discretion for local agencies, more devolution of powers from the centre could have taken place.

A review of local authority community strategies also revealed some shortcomings, with implications for partnerships in health and other areas (DCLG, 2008). There was much variation between councils in the amount of work undertaken on community strategies and in the level of resources allocated to them. There was some doubt about the value added by these strategies, and resources seem to have been reduced. Community strategies appeared to lose their importance as LAAs were introduced. However, community strategies were credited with enhancing partnership working, paving the way for more formal relationships through the LAAs.

There is limited evidence that specific programmes and initiatives led to an improvement in processes of partnership working or outcomes. HAZs allowed experimentation and learning between organizations and professionals (Bauld and McKenzie, 2007). They were also credited with establishing good foundations for long-term improvements in partnership working on health (Boydell and Rugkasa, 2007). Although there was some evidence of HAZs having a positive impact on health outcomes, this was not consistently the case (Smith, K. et al., 2009; Perkins et al., 2010), but they did have an impact on local agendas, raising the profile of health inequalities and the need to address the social determinants of health. It was also believed that HAZs stimulated public involvement. Some were concerned that this was tokenistic (Crawshaw et al., 2003). Even so, some HAZs made considerable efforts to promote genuine participation within a context of community development (see Chapter 5). HLCs were also credited with a number of achievements. They had some success in developing partnerships between the NHS and local government and with the voluntary sector (Hills et al., 2007). They engaged successfully with disadvantaged communities, helped people to adopt healthier lifestyles and involved people in planning and delivering services (Hills et al., 2007). However, as with HAZs, there was much variation. Some projects were very successful in building partnerships between local agencies and between public bodies and the community (see Bromley By Bow Centre, 2012), while others were less effective in this regard.

JSNAs were credited with improvements in joint working between councils and the NHS (Hughes, 2009; Local Government Information Unit, 2010). However, Hunter et al. (2011) identified problems with the compiling of JSNAs, including problems with the quality of data and the sharing of data between agencies. Research by the King's Fund found that JSNAs were rated as useful by local authorities but needed development and a stronger focus on priorities, and should include other relevant areas such as housing, employment and culture (Humphries et al., 2012). Many respondents wanted JSNAs to be more user-friendly, succinct and web-based, and therefore more useful and potentially more influential over commissioners. Other researchers found that despite significant progress in the quality of JSNAs between 2008 and 2010, key issues remained (Harding and Kane, 2011). This study found a cluster of high performers while others were lagging behind and had not got to grips with the JSNA process. Weaknesses that had to be addressed included ensuring that the required resources, expertise and audit skills were available, ensuring leadership and ownership of the JSNAs and linking with local health strategies, equipping JSNAs to lead commissioning and investment decisions, establishing their value to all parties, and strengthening accountability and public engagement.

It has long been acknowledged that NHS services should be commissioned on the basis of needs and with the aim of improving public health and well-being. Efforts to bring public health considerations into the commissioning process were made, but with little success. In practice, public health carried less weight than clinical considerations. This was illustrated by the 'raids' on public health budgets to other health services in the mid-2000s (Wanless, 2007). Furthermore, it was found that commissioners varied in the degree to which they reflected a public health ethos, incentivized prevention and prioritized investment in health and well-being (Marks et al., 2011).

Meanwhile, joint commissioning in public health remained underdeveloped. It moved more quickly in some areas (for example, children's services) than in others (Hunter et al., 2011). Joint appointments between the NHS and local government, particularly of local DPHs, have been identified as an important feature of partnership working in this field. For example, research by Hunter et al. (2011) revealed a 'near universal' view that joint DPH posts were effective. Joint DPH appointments were seen as a crucial bridge and facilitator between local authorities and PCTs, ensured that public health priorities were joined up strategically, helped to break down cultural divisions between organizations, and helped DPHs themselves to become more knowledgeable about the local authority/NHS context, enabling them to make better informed decisions. However, the effectiveness of such arrangements depended on many factors – including coherence of local policies and existing good relations between local agencies – and by itself did not guarantee effective partnership working (Hunter et al., 2010, 2011).

Partnership working on health may have been encouraged by programmes and reforms in other policy areas. For example, regeneration programmes were identified as stimulating partnership working in health. An evaluation of the New Deal for Communities found some positive health outcomes, although these could not be directly attributed to the programme (Smith, K. et al., 2009). Other relevant areas where the government sought to strengthen partnership working included health inequalities and children's health and well-being (explored in more detail in Boxes 3.1 and 3.2, respectively). In both cases, there was some evidence of improvements in joint working, but also some signs of continuing problems in both processes and – particularly in the case of health inequalities – some poor outcomes.

Box 3.2   Children's health and well-being

Policies on children's health and well-being introduced by New Labour were seen as providing a major stimulus to partnership working. For example, Sure Start, a programme aimed at supporting families with pre-school children, initially in the most deprived areas, sought to imbue a more collaborative approach between the NHS, local authorities and the voluntary sector in the provision of services for this client group, such as early education, health services, advice for parents and childcare. School-based health and well-being was another focus for the pursuit of a joined-up approach, notably through the Healthy Schools programme and the explicit recognition of the school's role in promoting the welfare of pupils.

Child safety and protection was yet another strand of policy in which interagency collaboration was emphasized. Following the Victoria Climbié case (Cm 5730, 2003), which highlighted key failings of interagency working in child protection, the *Every Child Matters* reforms were launched (Cm 5860, 2003). This agenda was driven by a designated minister for Children, Young People and Families, and later a new Department for Children, Schools and Families. Children's services authorities were created in local government with a brief to promote cooperation among all agencies with responsibilities in this field. These authorities were also charged with producing local plans for children and young people. Children's Trusts – multiagency arrangements for promoting children's welfare – and local safeguarding bodies were established. New duties to safeguard and promote the welfare of children were placed on agencies, including NHS bodies. Powers to create pooled budgets for children's services were also enacted. The various elements of children's welfare policy, along with initiatives to reduce child poverty, came together in a comprehensive Children's Plan, which further underlined the importance of collaborative working across agencies over a range of welfare issues (Cm 7280, 2007). This was followed by a Children and Young People's Health strategy, which reiterated the importance of partnership working in this particular field (Department for Children, Schools and Families and DH, 2009).

The outcome of these various initiatives was, on balance, positive, but with certain limitations. The Healthy Schools programme achieved key process objectives, in that key targets for recruiting schools to the scheme were met (75 per cent of schools by summer 2009). However, problems of implementation were identified, and it was found that schools varied in their commitment (OFSTED, 2006; Wicklander, 2006; Barnard et al., 2009). There was little evidence of impact on outcomes, apart from a small increase in participation in PE and sport, which was not uniform and may have been due to other policies that promoted increased physical activity.

Sure Start was credited with helping to improve partnership working at local level (Brown and Liddle, 2005; Gidley, 2007). However, much variation was apparent both in the quality of partnership working and in the leadership and management of Sure Start projects (Belsky et al., 2006). In the short term, Sure Start achieved positive outcomes in only five of the 14 child health and development outcomes identified (Melhuish et al., 2008). Doubts were expressed about the programme's ability to produce long-term changes (Kane, 2008). There was also disappointment that it failed to reach the most disadvantaged families and had a limited impact on health inequalities. However, Sure Start was popular with users and had a strong community and user involvement ethos (Brown and Liddle, 2005; Gustafson and Driver, 2005) even though constrained by professional power and top-down performance management (Myers et al., 2004; Gustafson and Driver, 2005; Children, School and Families Committee, 2010). Sure Start programmes made limited use of community development techniques to engage with local communities and users, and there were problems involving smaller voluntary and community organizations (Craig et al., 2007; see Chapter 6).

With regard to child protection legislation, there are difficulties in evaluating the impact of policies as they have been subject to continuous change. The partnerships arrangements established by *Every Child Matters* were reformed within a few years of being established, in the light of new child abuse scandals that exposed the shortcomings of the reforms (Lord Laming, 2009). Even before this occurred, it appeared that the new structures were struggling to overcome barriers to interagency working and improve outcomes (Audit Commission, 2008).

Although the evidence base for partnership working in public health is weak, much has been written about the factors that impede good joint working relationships in this field. These appear to be as follows:

■ *Reorganization and 'initiative-itis'.* Many have argued that partnership working has been inhibited by constant reorganization of the NHS and local government (McMurray, 2007; Hunter et al., 2011). Furthermore, the multiple initiatives to improve partnership working have often not been coordinated or planned within a coherent framework, and this has led to duplication, confusion and inconsistency (Health Committee, 2009; Perkins et al., 2010; Hunter et al., 2011). There has also been an overemphasis on short-term initiatives and 'quick wins' (Health Committee, 2009; Perkins et al., 2010).

■ *Insufficient resources.* Lack of resources, and arguments over who pays, can hamper partnership working (Perkins et al., 2010; Hunter et al., 2011). Public health partnership initiatives have in the past suffered from being deemed a low priority by both the NHS and local government (see Wanless, 2007). Funding for public health projects has often been short term and has not benefited from pooled budget arrangements to the same degree as social care (Audit Commission, 2009; Hunter et al., 2011).

■ *The dominance of the health and social care interface.* Some argue that partnership working between the NHS and local government has been dominated by social care issues and that this has been to the detriment of public health partnerships (Snape, 2004; Darlow et al., 2007). This may have been offset to a small extent, however, by a more preventive focus in relation to particular groups receiving social care (for example, preventing falls in elderly people, and suicides and self-harm in people with mental illness). Notably, however, the lack of integration between healthcare and social care continued to be a focus for criticism and still is today (Health Committee, 2012a; Wistow, 2012).

■ *Political, cultural and organizational factors.* Hunter et al. (2011) argue that barriers to partnership working in public health include resistance in local government (particularly among councillors) to cede territory to the NHS, different interpretations of the meaning of health and well-being between partners, and confusion about partnership responsibilities and roles. A failure to engage senior management in partnership arrangements is also problematic, as is not sharing information and good practice (Perkins et al., 2010). Lack of co-terminosity is also perceived as a problem (Perkins et al., 2010). Notably, in their study of health promotion partnerships, Jones and Barry (2011) found that trust, leadership and efficiency were the most important predictors of partnership synergy.

Another possible explanation for the limited effectiveness of partnerships in public health is that they have operated against the grain of other, arguably stronger, policies. These policies include those aimed at producing more competition and choice (choose and book, payment by results, Foundation Trusts, and private and voluntary sector provision). It is argued by some that these policies, pursued vigorously by the Labour government from 2000 onwards, undermined the ethos of collaboration that provides an essential basis for partnership working (Hunter et al., 2011).

Finally, much of the blame for the inadequacies of public health partnerships has been laid at the door of central government. It is often argued that NHS bodies and local councils often operate in silos because of national legislation, strategies and performance management frameworks, which are often not aligned (LGA, 2008). Moreover, both NHS and local government complain of mixed messages from central government departments (Hunter et al., 2011), indicative of poor coordination in central government on public health matters (Health Committee, 2001, 2009; Cabinet Office, 2007; Health Commission and Audit Commission, 2008). As noted earlier, much effort had been made to improve coordination within central government under both the Blair and Brown governments. These appear to have had some positive impact, although performance (across all policies and not just health) was described as variable in an Institute for Government report, which highlighted a key problem that lessons were not being systematically learned across central government (Parker et al., 2010). Prescriptions for further improvement made in this report included: fewer and clearer objectives for central government, better governance within central government departments with clearer responsibilities for delivering objectives, and stronger collaborative mechanisms and processes (including stronger incentives, explicit budgets, sharing of information and other resources, clearer responsibilities, and better performance management and appraisal systems to support collaboration).

Although central government policy coherence and support for partnership working is important, overemphasis on central initiatives can undermine local partnerships. Research by Hunter et al. (2011) found that partnership working was dominated by a 'top-down' approach that stifled local initiative. Those they interviewed agreed that partnerships worked better from the 'bottom up' than 'top down'. It was believed that, even within local partnerships and organizations, too much emphasis was placed on strategy and process. A disconnect was identified between the strategic level of partnership organizations and frontline services. This was characterized by poor vertical communication and information flows, and a lack of ownership of strategies and targets by those operating on the front line. Some respondents perceived tokenism at senior management level, coupled with a lack of understanding of the 'natural' propensity to form partner relationships at the frontline level. Moreover, the bureaucratic processes at strategic level were seen by some as posing a barrier to effective partnership working on the ground.

Partnerships in Scotland, Wales and Northern Ireland

Although there has always been some policy variation between different parts of the UK (Greer, 2009b), the advent of devolution in the late 1990s increased the potential for divergence in many areas, including health. Partnership working in health has been affected by devolution in four main respects. First, health and healthcare is an important area of devolved responsibility for the assemblies and parliaments of the devolved countries. Second, devolved responsibilities in areas related to public health, such as environment, transport and social policy, have also led to policy developments that affect public health partnership working. Third, under devolution, new structures of local governance have developed in Scotland, Wales and Northern Ireland, which have implications for health partnerships. Fourth, and considered in more detail in Chapter 5, different structures and processes of public and community engagement have also developed in these countries, compared with England, and these too have been relevant to partnership working in health.

Scotland

In Scotland, successive health strategies have emphasized public health and the importance of partnerships (Scottish Office, 1991, 1992; Cm 4269, 1999; Scottish Executive, 2000, 2003a, 2003b; Scottish Government, 2007a, 2007b). Although, as in other parts of the UK, a key focus of partnership has been upon integrating health and social care, there has been considerable effort north of the border to integrate health improvement within public sector planning. In 2002, new arrangements were introduced to enable NHS bodies and councils to pool budgets, mainly relating to social care. In 2003, local authorities were required to establish Community Planning Partnerships (CPPs) to deliver better and more joined-up public services. These include public and private sector bodies as well as community and voluntary sector representatives, including NHS bodies. CPPs draw up overarching community plans for their area and are also required to produce joint health improvement plans. They have a lead role on some health-related issues, notably health inequalities. In 2009, CPPs were given responsibility for Single Outcome Agreements for their area, which set out shared local objectives and outcomes, including health. A recent analysis by Audit Scotland (2013), however, found shortcomings in the way in which CPPs worked. In particular, CPPs were unable to demonstrate significant impact on outcomes and were not sufficiently clear about priorities. It also found that community planning had little impact on how resources were allocated. Moreover, governance was found to be poor, with member organizations (including health bodies) not being held to account for their performance.

Partnership working was included as an important component of programmes in specific fields of public health such as sexual health, cancer prevention, children's health and the prevention of coronary heart disease. In 2005, Community Health Partnerships (CHPs) were created to strengthen coordination between the NHS, local government and the voluntary sector. These statutory bodies, established within each health board and mostly aligned with local authority boundaries, aimed to integrate primary and acute services, bring together community-based health and social care, integrate children's services, promote closer working between the NHS and local authorities, improve health and reduce health inequalities. CHPs were also expected to engage with communities in their area. As CHPs were intended to be flexible in meeting local needs, there was little prescription about how they should operate (although some guidance was issued, for example on CHP membership and involving communities). Consequently, they varied considerably (Evans and Forbes, 2009; Ball et al., 2010; Watt et al., 2010; Audit Scotland, 2011). Some focused on integrating primary, community and secondary health services, while others were more geared to integrating health and social care (known as Community Health and Social Care Partnerships or Community Health and Care Partnerships). CHPs in their various forms were expected to involve key stakeholders among their membership (from the NHS, local authorities and the voluntary and community sectors), but governance and management structures varied.

Although flexibility had some benefits, for example in enabling the adoption of locally sensitive structures, serious questions were raised about the efficacy of CHPs (Watt et al., 2010; Audit Scotland, 2011). Shortcomings included confusion about their multiple roles, weak governance structures, poor accountability and a lack of influence on NHS and local government strategies. In particular, CHPs were unable to provide the kind of strong leadership needed to integrate services and strengthen partnership working. An in-depth study of staff in one CHP found that professional identities remained strong while partnership vision lacked clarity (Pate et al., 2010). Furthermore, Ball et al. (2010) found weaknesses in tackling cross-cutting issues and the alignment and pooling of budgets, although, on a more positive note, they found a number of areas of strength, including recognition by CHPs of common goals, and a need for partnership working, trust and leadership. This study also found that the inclusiveness of partnerships, in particular working with the voluntary sector, was rated highly by CHPs.

Concern was expressed about the duplication of efforts with other partnership initiatives and partnership bodies, notably, the CPPs' health and well-being brief, which overlaps significantly with the work of CHPs (Audit Scotland, 2011). In some local areas, this had been resolved by CHPs operating as the health and well-being 'arm' of CPPs. Other areas included CHP representatives on CPP bodies to improve coordination. But elsewhere there was little or no relationship between the CHP and the CPP (see also Audit Scotland, 2013). Other issues identified by Audit Scotland (2011) included problems with the sharing of information, and with monitoring the use of resources across health and social care. It did find, however, that progress had been made with sharing of premises. A further problem, noted by Watt et al. (2010), is that most CHPs found it difficult to work with GPs and also to some extent with clinicians in secondary care. More positively, Ball et al. (2010) found that health improvement, such as reducing death from preventable illness and reducing health inequalities, was a high priority for the CHPs they studied, although actual performance in this field was modest. Although there is evidence that some CHPs have been active in improving health in areas such as smoking cessation, obesity, alcohol and drug misuse, and in reducing health inequities, it is recognized that a stronger focus is needed on such issues (Watt et al., 2010).

Audit Scotland (2011) found considerable variation in public health performance indicators across CHP areas. On some indicators (drug- and alcohol-related hospital admissions and breastfeeding at eight weeks, for example), a majority of CHP areas experienced a deterioration in performance. On others (for example, smoking during pregnancy), the majority experienced an improvement. Variation was also found at the national level, where some indicators got worse (inequalities in heart disease deaths) while others improved (a slight reduction in inequalities in relation to low-birthweight babies). With regard to national outcome indicators of the effectiveness of health and social care collaboration, Audit Scotland (2011) found rising levels of delayed discharges from hospital in recent years (after a period of significant decline between 2002 and 2008) and an increase in multiple emergency admissions for older people.

Amid these concerns, the Scottish government announced in 2011 that CHP bodies would be replaced by Health and Social Care Partnerships, which would have a stronger focus on improving and integrating health and social care for adults, especially older people. These new bodies would have stronger joint accountability to NHS boards and local councils, and to ministers. It was also stated that professionals would have a greater role in service planning and promised additional legislation to facilitate service integration. Building on earlier efforts to develop an Integrated Resources Framework for health and social care, the government stated that, in future, NHS boards and councils would be required to produce integrated budgets. There would also be a greater emphasis on the shifting of resources to community-based provision, and on the achievement of joint outcomes.

Wales

In Wales, public health has been a stated priority since the late 1980s. The Welsh approach has emphasized the need to address the social and economic and environmental roots of ill health. A strong theme running through successive Welsh health strategy documents has been to invest resources in public health services and measures in order to produce 'health gain', sustained improvements in health and well-being, while reducing health inequalities (Welsh Office, 1989, 1998; National Assembly for Wales, 2001; Welsh Assembly Government, 2002, 2003a). Partnership working has been a key component of Welsh strategies and action plans. Initially, the focus was upon building 'healthy alliances' at local level, bringing together organizations with an interest in public health, such as NHS bodies, local authorities and the voluntary sector. This was bolstered by a statutory duty imposed on health boards and local authorities to work in partnership with each other and with other stakeholders. A requirement for the NHS and local councils to produce joint health, social care and well-being strategies for their area was also introduced. Incentives to promote partnership working were implemented, including additional funding for partnerships and pooled/delegated budgets between the NHS and local councils. It should be noted that partnership working in Wales was enhanced by the co-terminous boundaries of health boards and councils. However, a reorganization in 2009 that reduced the number of health boards to seven means that NHS boards are no longer co-terminous with individual local authorities (although each local authority area lies within the boundary of one health board).

Partnership working has been further encouraged by subsequent policy developments. The revised health strategy, *Designed for Life* (Welsh Assembly Government, 2005), reiterated the importance of partnership working in achieving public health objectives. A campaign to improve health in Wales, Health Challenge Wales, also acknowledged the importance of multiagency efforts. The latest public health strategy, *Our Healthy Future*, renews the commitment of the Welsh government to the improvement of health and well-being, and the reduction of health inequities (Welsh Assembly Government, 2009). The plan highlights the importance of health as a shared goal and a key focus for partnership working. Meanwhile, wider local government reforms in Wales have emphasized that health is a shared responsibility across local organizations and that these bodies must work together more effectively in partnership with each other (Welsh Assembly Government, 2006, 2007). New structures were introduced to facilitate this, including community strategy partnerships, which seek to bring together local strategies across traditional service boundaries. In addition, local service boards and local service agreements have been introduced in an effort to integrate planning, performance management and delivery across public service bodies.

Despite all these efforts, and examples of good practice in partnership working, it is clear that there is much scope for improvement (Wanless, 2003; Beecham Review, 2006; Entwhistle, 2006; NLIAH, 2009). Partners often have different perspectives, and partnerships have struggled to overcome this when seeking to address issues that cut across different policy and institutional agendas. In addition, the plethora of strategies and plans on public health, local governance and health have created some confusion, and one way forward is to ensure a better integration of policy at national level. It remains to be seen whether the 2009 reorganization of the NHS in Wales and the resulting loss of co-terminosity between health boards and local authorities has had detrimental effects on partnership working. Meanwhile, at the time of writing, the Welsh government is consulting on whether to place statutory duties on bodies to consider public health issues. Such a requirement, if enacted, could significantly strengthen the basis of partnerships in the field of health and well-being.

Northern Ireland

In Northern Ireland, strategies on health have strongly emphasized public health interventions and the importance of partnership working. In the late 1990s, public health targets were set across a range of issues, including the health of children and elderly people, where the importance of working across agencies was acknowledged as essential (DHSSNI, 1996, 1997). Subsequent strategies have continued to promote public health partnerships and joint planning (DHSSPS, 2002, 2004). Policy-makers in Northern Ireland have since devolution sought to develop a distinctive approach to public health and partnership working. Three key factors have shaped this response. Devolution powers initially granted in 1990 were suspended in 2002 due to a political crisis. Although these have since been restored, public health policy, like many other functions for which devolution was granted, was hindered by this suspension. Another factor has been the improved relationship between Northern Ireland and the Irish Republic, which has led to a stronger partnership approach on issues such as public health where there is much scope for collaboration. Notably, an all-Ireland Institute of Public Health was created in 1999 to promote even closer collaboration. A third factor has been the wider reform of public services and partnership arrangements in Northern Ireland. Due to the sectarian issues raised, this is been a highly political issue, and consequently reform has been slow. This has had a knock-on effect on local authority and NHS structures, and also on partnership arrangements on health matters.

Northern Ireland has a number of advantages for those seeking to improve partnership working. It has a relatively small population. The public sector reforms led to a smaller number of agencies and partnership bodies, which should be more conducive to joined-up working. It should also be noted that Northern Ireland also has a strong history of partnership working, for example on health and social care (having adopted integrated joint boards in the 1970s; Heenan and Birrell, 2006), and in its efforts to link social policy, regeneration and health agendas. Specific initiatives include HAZs, introduced in the late 1990s (similar to England), Investing for Health partnerships (to bring together local agencies to address socioeconomic and environmental determinants of health) and local health improvement plans. Also relevant to partnership working is Northern Ireland's considerable experience of community development and engagement in health and social policy, discussed further in Chapter 5.

Conclusion

The New Labour governments made a clear effort to improve partnership working both in general and in the area of public health and well-being. The healthcare and social care interface remained an important aspect of joint working and continued to dominate the health partnership agenda, although arguably not as overwhelmingly as before. Notably, even in health and social care, problems in getting different agencies to collaborate persisted. As Wistow (2012, p. 109) noted, 'much has been promised but little delivered'. The lessons from this arena are important. Wistow identifies fundamental barriers to integration: that responsibilities are based on the skills of providers and not on the needs of users, and that organizational forms are based on separation rather than interdependence (with the NHS and local government being based on different principles). He argues that a major flaw in policy has been the effort to bridge parallel organizations rather than interweave their mainstream processes. One possible way forward lies in joining together commissioning processes more effectively, for example by a single commissioning process (with a single commissioner responsible) for health, care and other services (such as housing) for particular client groups such as the elderly (Health Committee, 2012a). An even more radical approach would be to bring health and social care under one body, namely local government (as indeed has been suggested in the past – see Chapter 1).

It is difficult to assess the various initiatives on partnership working on health and well-being introduced by New Labour. Few reforms and projects were properly evaluated, and when they were there was insufficient emphasis on outcomes. Important lessons – both positive and negative – were not learned. New initiatives were introduced before previous ones had been fully evaluated. In addition, differences between different parts of the UK provided much scope for lesson-drawing, but this was not exploited. The evidence available suggests that the quality and effectiveness of partnership working in this field varied considerably, with some good practice and more progress in some specific areas (both geographical and policy areas) than others. However, the overall impact, given the amount of effort involved, was disappointing. Indeed, there were negative effects arising from partnership initiatives, including short-termism, an attempt to create technical solutions to what were actually political problems, centralization and weakened accountability.

4 Partnerships and the Coalition government

Introduction

This chapter examines the main changes and continuities in public health policy since 2010, under the Conservative–Liberal Democrat Coalition government led by David Cameron, and their impact on partnership working. After outlining the main features of the Coalition's reforms, the chapter focuses on the role of new local partnership bodies, Health and Wellbeing Boards. The chapter also features an analysis of multidisciplinary and interprofessional working, an important aspect of partnership working that is being addressed by the Coalition (and which has also been considered by previous governments).

The Cameron government's health reforms

The majority party in the Coalition government, the Conservatives, had proposed reforms of both the NHS and public health while in opposition. Their NHS policies emphasized the importance of choice and competition in healthcare, with alternative providers being allowed to provide NHS-funded services, greater empowerment of professionals, particularly in the process of commissioning services for patients, and more freedom for local bodies to make decisions about planning and services, with less emphasis on central targets (Conservative Party, 2007, 2009, 2010a). The Conservatives broadly agreed with many of the reforms introduced by New Labour and did not openly support a reorganization of the NHS structure at this time, their emphasis being instead on changing processes and improving outcomes.

With regard to public health, the Conservatives believed that there should be a stronger focus on improving health and reducing health inequalities, and a greater emphasis on prevention of illness (Conservative Research Department, 2007; Conservative Party, 2010b). They stated their intention to rename the Department of Health as the Department of *Public* Health, with a stronger coordinating role across government (although this idea was not taken forward). The Conservatives proposed a restructuring of public health, enabling local bodies, Primary Care Trusts (PCTs) and local authorities to decide on local priorities and how funding should be allocated. They also suggested a ring-fenced budget for public health, and additional resources for areas with high health needs and for those achieving health improvements. Other proposals included greater voluntary efforts by business to contribute towards health improvement (see Chapter 7), an expanded role for GPs and other primary care professionals in public health, and specific action on issues such as binge drinking and obesity.

The Liberal Democrats, the junior partner in the Coalition, also wanted to see more devolution of decision-making in the NHS, although they placed more emphasis on greater local accountability and democracy (Liberal Democrats, 2008, 2010). They specifically urged substantial cuts in central health bureaucracy (including the Department of Health) and the abolition of Strategic Health Authorities (SHAs). The Liberal Democrats argued that health and social care should be integrated into a seamless service. They also supported action on key public health problems such as health inequalities, smoking, alcohol and obesity, and backed greater incentives for GPs to prevent illness.

So there was a considerable overlap between the two parties' health policies before they entered government. In an attempt to create a more coherent set of aims and priorities for the Coalition, a programme was agreed (HM Government, 2010a). A total of 54 commitments in this programme were health-related (28 related to the NHS, 21 to public health and five to social care). Specific commitments included increases in health spending in real terms year on year, a cessation of 'top-down reorganizations', a reduction in NHS administration and health quangos, strengthening of the power of GPs in commissioning, allowance for directly elected members of PCTs, the creation of an independent NHS board to allocate resources and provide commissioning guidelines, and greater involvement of independent and voluntary service providers in the NHS. With regard to public health, commitments included greater control for local communities over public health budgets, linking payments to health outcomes, giving greater incentives to GPs to tackle public health problems, exploring ways of improving access to preventive healthcare for those people living in disadvantaged areas, and policies to tackle alcohol and drug abuse.

However, when the government's NHS Reforms were outlined in a White Paper, *Equity and Excellence: Liberating the NHS* in July 2010 (Cm 7881, 2010), there was much surprise at the radical nature of the reorganization proposed therein, particularly given the commitment to avoid top-down reorganizations. The White Paper heralded the abolition of PCTs and SHAs and the transfer of commissioning functions to local consortia of GPs. At national level, an NHS Commissioning Board (since renamed as NHS England) would be created to issue guidelines and directly commission some services (for example, primary care and some specialized services). The board would implement NHS priorities set by the Secretary of State for Health, who would in future set a policy framework rather than intervene directly in the NHS. All NHS Trusts would become Foundation Trusts, and the NHS would be opened to outside suppliers, the new market being regulated by the current Foundation Trust regulator, Monitor. Although the key focus was on the NHS, the White Paper had important implications for public health services. First, many of the services to be commissioned by NHS England and the GP consortia had public health implications (for example, primary care services and some disease prevention and health promotion services). The White Paper also proposed important changes in the structure of public health – namely the transfer of key public health responsibilities and functions to local authorities, and the creation of a national public health service to integrate existing health improvement and health protection expertise. Public health policy was further developed in a second White Paper, *Healthy Lives, Healthy People*, later the same year (Cm 7985, 2010). The key public health policies of the Coalition are listed in Box 4.1.

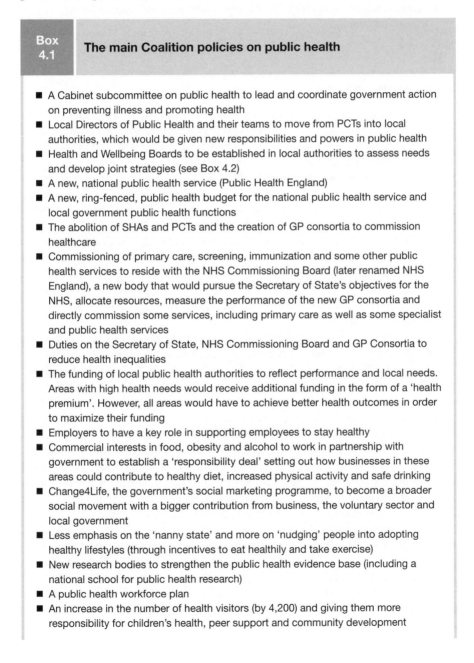

Box 4.1 **The main Coalition policies on public health**

- A Cabinet subcommittee on public health to lead and coordinate government action on preventing illness and promoting health
- Local Directors of Public Health and their teams to move from PCTs into local authorities, which would be given new responsibilities and powers in public health
- Health and Wellbeing Boards to be established in local authorities to assess needs and develop joint strategies (see Box 4.2)
- A new, national public health service (Public Health England)
- A new, ring-fenced, public health budget for the national public health service and local government public health functions
- The abolition of SHAs and PCTs and the creation of GP consortia to commission healthcare
- Commissioning of primary care, screening, immunization and some other public health services to reside with the NHS Commissioning Board (later renamed NHS England), a new body that would pursue the Secretary of State's objectives for the NHS, allocate resources, measure the performance of the new GP consortia and directly commission some services, including primary care as well as some specialist and public health services
- Duties on the Secretary of State, NHS Commissioning Board and GP Consortia to reduce health inequalities
- The funding of local public health authorities to reflect performance and local needs. Areas with high health needs would receive additional funding in the form of a 'health premium'. However, all areas would have to achieve better health outcomes in order to maximize their funding
- Employers to have a key role in supporting employees to stay healthy
- Commercial interests in food, obesity and alcohol to work in partnership with government to establish a 'responsibility deal' setting out how businesses in these areas could contribute to healthy diet, increased physical activity and safe drinking
- Change4Life, the government's social marketing programme, to become a broader social movement with a bigger contribution from business, the voluntary sector and local government
- Less emphasis on the 'nanny state' and more on 'nudging' people into adopting healthy lifestyles (through incentives to eat healthily and take exercise)
- New research bodies to strengthen the public health evidence base (including a national school for public health research)
- A public health workforce plan
- An increase in the number of health visitors (by 4,200) and giving them more responsibility for children's health, peer support and community development

- Children's centres to continue but must work more closely with the private and voluntary sectors
- Measures to reduce binge drinking and underage drinking (such as a ban on the sale of below-cost-price alcohol, increased penalties for serving underage drinkers, and stronger licensing controls on outlets and hours of sale)
- A consultation on measures to require tobacco to be sold in plain packaging
- Further initiatives promised on specific public health problems, such as alcohol, tobacco and obesity

Public health reforms

Compared with the reorganization of the NHS, the public health measures were relatively uncontroversial. Indeed, there was much support for the broad thrust of policy, in particular the transfer of local leadership in public health to local authorities (that is, unitary authorities, county councils and London boroughs, all of which have social services responsibilities). This would entail a transfer from PCTs (abolished in 2013) of the Directors of Public Health (DPHs) and their public health teams. In theory, this would strengthen local authorities' strategic role in public health. This was acknowledged as important in the light of the 'place-shaping' role of local authorities (see Chapter 3). Embedding public health teams in local authorities also raised the prospect of greater collaboration with other local authority departments and agencies that were providing care and support and/or could influence the causes of ill health (for example, adult social services, children's services, education, planning, transport, housing, leisure services and environmental health).

There were, however, some critical voices. Some doubted that transferring responsibilities and staff would necessarily strengthen the public health function (Hunter et al., 2011; Maryon-Davis, 2011; McKee et al., 2011; Public Health for the NHS, 2012). Organizational changes were seen as a threat to existing partnerships, causing dislocation and disruption. There was also concern about the capacity of local government to take on new public health roles. Doubts were expressed that the amount of money available to local authorities would be sufficient for the task. It was acknowledged that, in the prevailing adverse economic climate, securing additional resources for public health from other local government budgets would be difficult. Indeed, despite the 'ring-fencing' of public health budgets, it was feared that councils might redesignate other spending as 'public health', diverting resources to other priorities (McKee et al., 2011).

Another problem was that key public health functions would remain outside the control of local public health departments. In areas with two-tier local government authorities (county and district councils), some functions, including environmental health and housing resided with the latter, and therefore outside the remit of the public health team's employing authority (Health Committee, 2011a). As discussed later, there was mounting criticism that the contribution of district councils was not fully acknowledged by the reforms.

Moreover, important public health functions remained in the NHS. The government intended that consortia of GP practices (later reformulated as Clinical Commissioning Groups [CCGs]) would replace PCTs, taking over their planning and commissioning role for secondary services. GPs and other primary care providers would continue to provide public health services, such as immunization, child health surveillance, health promotion and screening. To complicate matters even further, commissioning for primary care services and some public health services (including screening, immunization, public health services for people in prison and other places of detention, sexual assault services and – until 2015 – public health services for children under five years of age) was given to NHS England. In some cases, strategic, commissioning and service responsibilities for a particular field were divided among several different bodies. The Health Committee (2011a, p. 72) noted that there was a danger of 'a lack of coordination and cohesion in public health services' (a point later reiterated by the Communities and Local Government Committee, 2013).

There was also concern about variations in services across different local areas. The government, keen to emphasize local discretion, identified only a few functions that local authorities must provide (so-called 'mandated services'): the national child measurement programme, public health advice to the NHS, sexual health services, health protection, and NHS health checks for people aged 40–74. (The government intended to mandate the child health programme for those aged 5–19 but did not implement it at this time.)

Changes to the Coalition's plans

The government's public health reforms were included alongside its NHS reorganization plans in the Health and Social Care Bill introduced in January 2011. As the bill moved through its early Parliamentary stages, criticism intensified, most of it aimed at the NHS reorganization. These plans were attacked by professional organizations and pressure groups, by Parliament and from within the government itself. Indeed, the Liberal Democrats, although 'signed up' to the reforms, called for fundamental changes at their conference in March 2011. In the face of these pressures, the government agreed to 'pause' the legislative process. This provided an opportunity to consult further on the legislation.

The NHS Future Forum was established, drawn from health and social care professions, management, local authorities, the voluntary sector and patients' and carers' groups. It reported in June 2011 with recommendations to modify the reforms, several of which were relevant to public health and partnership working (NHS Future Forum, 2011a). A key theme of these recommendations was that there should be effective multiprofessional involvement in the GP commissioning consortia. The Future Forum also stated that consortia must publish board papers and minutes, meet in public, have effective independent representation to protect against conflicts of interest and take on functions only when they were capable of doing so. It argued that commissioning be strengthened to better integrate services across health, social care and public health, recommending that commissioning consortia be responsible for a defined geographical area and population, and that their boundaries must wherever possible avoid crossing local authority boundaries.

The government's plan to create local Health and Wellbeing Boards (see Box 4.2 later in the chapter) was seen as having huge potential to generate service integration and improvements in population health. But the Future Forum wished to see more cooperation between the different local bodies involved. It supported stronger powers for Health and Wellbeing Boards to hold commissioners of health and social care services to account if their commissioning plans were not in line with joint health and well-being strategies (see below). In addition, the Future Forum was clear that independent public health expertise must be provided at every level of the system. It endorsed the duties placed on NHS bodies to reduce health inequalities, but warned that these needed to be translated into practical action. Finally, it stated that there should be greater public involvement in local health strategies, and that patient and public involvement in general should be strengthened (discussed further in Chapter 5).

The government responded by rebadging GP consortia as CCGs, with a wider membership including other clinicians and lay people. It conceded that NHS England and CCGs must draw on public health expertise when undertaking their functions. CCGs' responsibility for local residents was to some extent clarified, to include people registered with general practices that formed a CCG, as well as residents not registered with any general practice outside a CCG's area. An additional responsibility on CCGs to arrange emergency and urgent care for all people in their particular area was also introduced, along with powers to amend their responsibilities with regard to other specific population groups.

The government also sought to place greater emphasis on integration, through additional duties on NHS England and by strengthening Health and Wellbeing Boards, in ways discussed at length below. It also accepted a number of other amendments relevant to partnership working, including strengthening requirements to reduce health inequalities (intended as a key focus for local partnerships). The bill was amended to require CCGs to report on progress in reducing health inequalities related to access to healthcare and associated health outcomes. NHS England was given powers to issue guidance and to give financial incentives to CCGs to reduce health inequalities. Progress on reducing health inequalities was included in NHS England's performance assessment of CCGs. In addition, both NHS England and the Secretary of State for Health were given additional responsibilities to report on the progress of the NHS in reducing health inequalities. It was pointed out that this represented a narrow view of health inequalities, confined to inequalities in healthcare (Health Committee, 2011a). However, the Department of Health clarified that the Secretary of State's duties to reduce health inequalities applied to public health services as well as healthcare (Cm 8290, 2012).

A further issue raised was that local authorities appeared not have an equivalent duty to reduce health inequalities. The Department of Health responded by stating this it was unnecessary to include this in the bill because local authorities would be bound by a public health outcomes framework that included the reduction of health inequalities and by the provisions of the Equality Act 2010 (which seeks to prevent public authorities from discriminating against certain groups). This was confirmed by a ministerial reply to a Parliamentary Question: 'local authorities must have regard to reducing inequalities when commissioning public health services. The NHS and public health outcomes frameworks will be used to monitor progress' (Northover, 2013).

Another key area of partnership attracted attention from critics. There were fears that the new public health and NHS structures would be a recipe for poor coordination of emergency preparedness, such as for a bioterrorist attack or a serious outbreak of infectious disease (Health Committee, 2011a; Public Health for the NHS, 2012). The government allocated various responsibilities and duties of cooperation (to Public Health England – see Box 4.1, NHS England, the CCGs and local authorities). NHS England was required to ensure that CCGs were prepared in case of emergencies. Responsibilities were placed on NHS England, CCGs and service providers to have plans for such eventualities. Further guidance was promised that would clarify the roles of Public Health England, NHS England and local authorities in the context of specified local partnership arrangements (DH, 2012e).

This led to the establishment of Local Health Resilience Partnerships (LHRPs), bringing together health sector organizations in order to coordinate, plan and facilitate joint working. LHRPs are co-chaired by a lead public health director (from one of the upper-tier or unitary local authorities in the area) and a director responsible for emergency preparedness (drawn from NHS England's local area team). LHRPs are co-terminous with Local Resilience Forums (the partnership bodies responsible for coordinating multiagency plans and responses to emergencies). In addition, a commitment was made to ensure that regional public health structures (in the new system, the regional 'hubs' of Public Health England) would be co-terminous with NHS England regional structures and the regional resilience organizations of the Department for Communities and Local Government. Although this provided some reassurance, concern about a lack of clarity about responsibilities during health emergencies remained (Communities and Local Government Committee, 2013).

Other developments affecting public health partnerships

The government conceded a number of other changes that looked likely to strengthen public health functions and coordination. Its initial plan was to create Public Health England as a body within the Department of Health. However, amid concerns (including those expressed by the Future Forum and the Commons' Health Committee) that this could undermine the independence of public health advisory functions, the government decided to establish it as a non-departmental public body. DPHs were added to the list of statutory chief officers under the Local Government and Housing Act 1989, giving them similar status to Directors of Adult Social Services and Directors of Children's Services. This was in response to fears that DPHs might lack the clout needed to ensure that public health was a priority for their employing council. A further change was reflected in a series of amendments that required local authorities to have regard to statutory guidance issued by the Health Secretary on the appointment, termination of employment, terms and conditions, and management of DPHs. Provision was also made for similar guidance regarding other public health specialists employed by local authorities.

Meanwhile a range of other measures not contained in the Health and Social Care Bill had implications for future public health strategy and partnership working. The government's Localism Act (2011) contained five key measures: rights to give community organizations a chance to bid to take over land and buildings; neighbourhood planning, which allowed local communities to shape local development plans; measures to devolve housing decisions to the local level; measures to enable the transfer of public functions to local level; and a general power of competence giving councils greater freedom to take on additional functions in order to improve services and improve their local area. Coupled with the transfer of public health functions to local government, this Act held the potential for an expansion of community-based action on health and well-being.

The Coalition government abolished Government Offices for the Region (GORs), which managed the process of Local Area Agreements (LAAs), discussed in Chapter 3. LAAs were also abolished, along with Comprehensive Area Assessment (CAA). These policies had been introduced by New Labour with the aim of breaking down silos and institutional barriers between local agencies. Although not entirely successful, they were credited with bringing about some improvements in the context of partnership working. However, it should not be assumed that by reversing these policies, partnership working was necessarily damaged. As Hunter et al. (2011) argued, 'top-down' approaches to partnership can inhibit more flexible forms of partnership at the frontline or operational level.

Subsequent developments indicated that the new government was willing to build on some of its predecessors' policies on partnership working, especially those that sought to pool budgets at local level, such as Total Place and participatory budgeting. The Coalition introduced a programme of community budgets. These schemes enabled the pooling of funds from central government for tackling particular problems, initially focusing on 'troubled' families with complex needs. In addition, a pilot programme of Whole-Place Community budgets was established in four areas (Greater Manchester, Essex, Cheshire and Chester, and West London). These areas sought to pool budgets to address different challenges including: welfare dependency, skills gaps and workless households; the need to integrate health and social care and support people with chronic conditions; and tackling domestic abuse and antisocial behaviour. Ten neighbourhood-level community budget pilots were also established to give residents a greater say in local services. It is expected that, under such schemes, councils will work together with local communities, the voluntary sector and other public sector agencies to meet local priorities. If these programmes are extended as envisaged, this is likely to bring stronger financial incentives for agencies to work together on common issues within defined local areas. The disadvantage, however, is that the emphasis on the local level may lead to a lack of strategic vision, and duplication may arise. Another potential problem is that the smaller localities may have insufficient capacity and resources to deal with large-scale or challenging issues. A related initiative, City Deals, involves central government devolving budgets to individual local authorities or clusters of local authorities to enable them to develop local economies and infrastructure. This is also expected to strengthen partnership working not just between local authorities but between different parts of the public sector and between the public and private sectors.

Although such initiatives to some extent continued the previous government's approach, the Coalition indicated that partnerships would in future be even more inclusive with regard to the non-state sector. The emphasis upon voluntary efforts to improve health, in the context of the government's encouragement of 'the Big Society', signalled a greater role for voluntary and community organizations in partnership working (see Chapter 6). Similarly, the government's endorsement of employer-led initiatives in health promotion and its pursuit of responsibility deals with commercial interests implied a greater partnership role for business (see Chapter 7).

Health and Wellbeing Boards

One of the most significant changes regarding public health partnership working was the creation of local Health and Wellbeing Boards, and this section explores these in some depth. Health and Wellbeing Boards were proposed in response to pressures for a greater integration of services across healthcare, public health and social care, and by demands that local authorities have a greater say in healthcare. It appears that the specific proposal was born out of a deal within the Coalition, in which a previous agreement between the parties to introduce direct elections for PCTs was dropped (following the decision to abolish these bodies) in return for a greater coordinating role in health for local authorities (Timmins, 2012).

Coordinating bodies on health and well-being had already been established informally in many areas prior to this. Their creation had been stimulated by the need to agree the health dimensions of LAAs, fulfil statutory requirements to produce a Joint Strategic Needs Assessment (JSNA) and improve partnership working as part of the World Class Commissioning initiative (see Chapter 3). Initially, the Coalition wanted Health and Wellbeing Boards to take on the scrutiny function of local authorities, but following concerns that this would conflate strategic management, partnership working and scrutiny, and would bring the independence of scrutiny into question, it was decided not to pursue this course (and, as we saw in Chapter 3, scrutiny functions have also been reformed). The Coalition was also open on the question of whether Health and Wellbeing Boards should be statutory bodies. It eventually decided to establish them as a statutory committee within unitary and upper-tier local authorities.

Following the passage of the Health and Social Care Act 2012, Health and Wellbeing Boards were given functions and powers, and duties were placed on other bodies with regard to them. These are summarized in Box 4.2.

Box 4.2	Functions, duties and powers of Health and Wellbeing Boards and other relevant bodies

- Health and Wellbeing Boards are required to encourage those bodies arranging for the provision of health and social care services to work closely together and in an integrated manner in the improvement of health and well-being of people in the area
- They are also required to advise, assist and support the use of existing legal powers to pool and delegate budgets
- They may also encourage those arranging for the provision of health-related services (those which affect health but which are not considered to be health and social care services, such as housing) to work closely with themselves and with health and social care services
- Health and Wellbeing Boards lead the development of the JSNA and Joint Health and Wellbeing Strategy (JHWS) in their areas. JSNAs were introduced in later years of the Labour government (see Chapter 3) and are a joint statutory responsibility of CCGs (previously PCTs) and local authorities. The JHWS, covering healthcare, social care and public health, is based on the JSNA (and, like the JSNA, is a joint and equal statutory responsibility of local authorities and CCGs exercised through Health and Wellbeing Boards)
- Health and Wellbeing Boards must be involved in the preparation and revision of CCG commissioning plans in their area and must be consulted on whether drafts take proper account of their JHWS
- CCG commissioning plans must contain a statement from the relevant Health and Wellbeing Boards on their consistency with the JHWS. Also, a Health and Wellbeing Board can inform NHS England and the CCG if it believes that the final commissioning plan does not reflect the JHWS
- Health and Wellbeing Boards may provide advice to NHS England on the authorization of CCGs (the government accepted the principle that authorized CCG boundaries must not normally cross local authority boundaries – that is, they may only do so with good reason)
- CCGs have a statutory duty to work in partnership with local authorities and vice versa. There is a general duty of cooperation on matters of health and welfare, and now a specific duty on CCGs to cooperate with Health and Wellbeing Boards in the exercise of their functions
- NHS England must include in its assessments an analysis of the extent to which CCGs have had regard to the JSNA and JHWS. Health and Wellbeing Boards must be consulted by NHS England in its annual assessment of the performance of CCGs regarding how they contribute to the delivery of the JHWS
- Each CCG's annual report must review its contribution to the JHWS, and each relevant Health and Wellbeing Board must be consulted on this
- Local authorities must have regard to the JSNA and JHWS when commissioning services, and the Health and Wellbeing Board can give an opinion on whether the local authority has discharged its duty
- NHS England must have regard to the JSNA and JHWS when commissioning services for that area
- The Health and Wellbeing Board must consult and involve people who live or work in their area (as well as the local healthwatch – see Chapter 5) in the preparation of the JSNA and JHWS

- Health and Wellbeing Boards, like local authorities and NHS bodies, are themselves subject to scrutiny
- In preparing the JSNA and JHWS, the Health and Wellbeing Board must have regard to guidance issued by the Secretary of State for Health. In addition, when preparing the JSNA, it is required to have regard to the Secretary of State for Health's 'Mandate' (the annual statement of objectives for NHS England, along with any requirements and a statement of financial resources available to the NHS)
- Health and Wellbeing Boards can request information from their members in order to enable them to perform their functions
- Local authorities can delegate any local authority function except scrutiny to a Health and Wellbeing Board
- Health and Wellbeing Boards are free to establish subcommittees and delegate functions to them
- Health and Wellbeing Boards are exempt from standard requirements on local authority committees in that non-elected members may vote and the political composition of the membership is left to local discretion
- Health and Wellbeing Boards may make arrangements for any of their functions to be exercised jointly or by a joint subcommittee. Two or more Health and Wellbeing Boards may decide to work together to produce a JSNA and JHWS for their combined geographical area
- Health and Wellbeing Boards are also responsible for pharmaceutical needs assessments (which are important in making decisions about NHS-funded services in local community pharmacies and when deciding whether new pharmacies are needed in the area)

The required membership of a Health and Wellbeing Board – set out in the Health and Social Care Act 2012 – consists of the DPH, the Director of Children's Services, the Director of Adult Social Services, representatives from CCGs in the area, at least one councillor (and/or an elected mayor in authorities that have adopted this arrangement) and a member of the local healthwatch organization (to represent patients and the public – discussed further in Chapter 5). A further requirement is that a representative of NHS England must sit on the board when local authorities are drawing up their JSNA and Joint Health and Wellbeing Strategy (JHWS). In addition, others may be co-opted to the Health and Wellbeing Board at the local authority's discretion, or by the board itself.

There was much interest in the initial proposals to establish Health and Wellbeing Boards. The majority of eligible local authorities created 'shadow' boards before the legislation was passed. Despite this enthusiasm, there was concern that the new bodies would not have sufficient powers to ensure compliance with the JHWS (Maryon-Davis, 2011; NHS Future Forum, 2011a). This led to a significant strengthening of the relevant clauses of the bill during its Parliamentary stages. In the original bill, a duty was imposed on commissioning bodies to 'have regard to' the JSNA and the JHWS. The GP consortia (as originally conceived) were expected to cooperate with the Health and Wellbeing Boards in the exercise of their functions and in particular to contribute to the JSNA and JHWS. Moreover, each consortium was required to consult local Health and Wellbeing Boards about its commissioning plan and the extent to which it reflected the JSNA and JHWS. The Health and Wellbeing Board was in turn permitted to comment on the commissioning plans of the GP consortium in its area and have its opinion included as a statement in the final commissioning plan. In addition, the government promised that Health and Wellbeing Boards would be able to notify the local authority and/or NHS England if they believed that commissioning plans did not have sufficient regard to the local JSNA or JHWS.

Following the reconsideration of the bill, these elements were strengthened further. Local authority and CCG duties to have regard to the JSNA and JHWS were widened to cover any of their functions, not just those deemed to have a significant effect on needs. Health and Wellbeing Boards were given a closer involvement in the development of commissioning plans, rather simply being consulted. CCGs were now required to report on their contribution to the JHWS and consult Health and Wellbeing Boards on this. NHS England would now have to review how well CCGs were performing on their duty to have regard to the JSNA and JHWS, and would have to consult each Health and Wellbeing Board when conducting this. Demands that Health and Wellbeing Boards be able to veto CCG commissioning plans were not, however, conceded, although the boards were given a role in the authorization of CCGs and could object to their proposed boundaries. Another important amendment affecting Health and Wellbeing Boards was that they had to have regard to the NHS Mandate and also any guidance from the Secretary of State when formulating the JHWS. The bill was also changed to place an obligation on Health and Wellbeing Boards to involve the local healthwatch, and people who live and work in the area, in preparing their strategies.

During the passage of the legislation, concern was also expressed about the composition of Health and Wellbeing Boards, as well as confusion about responsibilities and a lack of accountability in the proposed joint working arrangements. The Health Committee (2011b) found the processes 'unnecessarily bureaucratic' and recommended that Health and Wellbeing Boards be dropped from the legislation. It called for the responsibility for the JSNA, the JHWS and the promotion of integrated working to be shared jointly by the NHS Commissioning Board (NHS England), GP commissioners (CCGs) and local authorities. The committee also recommended that, in place of Health and Wellbeing Boards, statutory governance arrangements for local health commissioning bodies should prescribe that their governing boards include an elected local authority member and a professional social care representative, as well as a public health expert, an elected councillor (or directly elected mayor), a nursing representative and a representative of hospital medicine. The government accepted the recommendations to include a nursing and a hospital representative on the CCG board, but rejected the others. Indeed, it specifically prohibited councillors from being members of these bodies. This decision has been criticized for weakening accountability and partnership working (Communities and Local Government Committee, 2013).

In a further criticism, the Commons' Health Committee (2011a), while acknowledging that the government had made significant changes to the bill, expressed concern that district councils in county areas were not automatically represented on Health and Wellbeing Boards (although they now had a right to be involved in the JSNA, strengthening their existing consultation rights introduced in the 2007 Local Government and Public Involvement in Health Act). An attempt to amend the Health and Social Care bill to ensure that district councillors had a seat on Health and Wellbeing Boards in county areas was unsuccessful. There remained a broader concern about how the boards would bring together the various parties, in particular to integrate services, especially given the lack of statutory powers and incentives available and the division between strategy and delivery in counties with two-tier councils (Kuznetsova, 2012). Some Health and Wellbeing Boards, however, made a clear effort to bring district councils into the fold (see Communities and Local Government Commitee, 2013). The government responded by strengthening its statutory guidance (see below), urging county councils to work with districts on JHWS even though this was not required by the Health and Social Care Act 2012 (see DH, 2013a).

The early impact of Health and Wellbeing Boards

The Coalition's health policy documents since the White Papers on the NHS and public health have continued to emphasize the importance of partnership, service integration and the role of Health and Wellbeing Boards. The NHS Commissioning Framework 2012–13 identified partnership working as important and highlighted the key role of Health and Wellbeing Boards in integrating services and overseeing local strategies across public health, social care and healthcare (DH, 2011b). The NHS Mandate (DH, 2012a) placed an emphasis on integrated services and a more joined-up experience for users. In addition, NHS England was given a role to drive and coordinate efforts to overcome barriers to joint working and to make partnership working successful. Its planning guidance for the NHS emphasized the importance of service integration and the need for NHS commissioners to work with Health and Wellbeing Boards and others to prevent premature mortality and improve care for people with long-term conditions (NHS National Commissioning Board, 2012). This also referred to the importance of Health and Wellbeing Boards in determining and overseeing local priorities and holding commissioners to account.

To guide and support the early development of Health and Wellbeing Boards, several documents were produced. These emerged from various consultation and development activities, including a national learning network for Health and Wellbeing Boards (funded by the Department of Health and supported by a range of bodies including the NHS Confederation, the Royal Society for Public Health and the Local Government Association) and stakeholder workshops. One of these documents set out operating principles for Health and Wellbeing Boards (NHS Confederation et al., 2011) as follows: to provide collective leadership to improve health and well-being across the local authority area; to enable shared decision-making and ownership of decisions in an open and transparent way; to achieve democratic legitimacy and accountability, and empower local people to take part in decision-making; to address health inequalities by ensuring that quality, consistency and comprehensive health and local government services were commissioned and delivered in the area; and to identify key priorities for health and local government commissioning and develop clear plans for how commissioners could make the best use of their combined resources to improve health and well-being outcomes. The document also identified in relation to each area what success might look like, and formulated specific questions to prompt boards to put these principles into practice (for example: Are there clear lines of accountability? Are health and well-being outcomes improving and health inequalities reducing? Do health and well-being partners work well together or are they operating individually?).

Another document set out operating principles for the JSNA and JHWS (NHS Confederation et al., 2012a): to review and learn from previous JSNAs (and previous local strategies); to agree the vision and scope of the JSNA and JHWS; to build a comprehensive picture of local needs and assets (including the skills, networks and resources of the community); and to enable stakeholder involvement throughout the process, including local authority departments, district councils, service providers, the voluntary and community sectors, and the wider public; to identify strategic priorities, including integration; and to influence commissioning plans and monitor outcomes. Other topics covered in documents produced by this collaboration included support and resources for health and well-being groups (NHS Confederation et al., 2012b), improving population health (NHS Confederation et al., 2012c) and encouraging integrated working to improve services (NHS Confederation et al., 2012d).

In addition, draft statutory guidance on the JSNA and JHWS was issued for consultation (DH, 2012b). The final version appeared in 2013 (DH, 2013a). This set out the responsibilities of Health and Wellbeing Boards in greater detail and clarified a number of matters raised by stakeholders. In short, the guidance re-emphasized the importance of local ownership of JSNAs and JHWSs, with the key aim of developing local evidence-based priorities for commissioning to improve health and well-being and reduce inequalities. Local flexibility was emphasized, for example in the timing and format of JSNA and JHWS documents. The guidance made it clear that Health and Wellbeing Boards should consider wider factors that impinge on health and well-being and specified areas including, for example, air quality, access to green space, employment, climate change, community safety, transport and housing. The document also sought to clarify their powers to request information (and duties of other bodies to respond). It also covered some accountability issues (for example, how the boards could raise matters with NHS England and local authorities in situations where they believed commissioning plans did not have sufficient regard to JSNAs and JHWSs). The guidance elaborated on partnership working, emphasizing the need for Health and Wellbeing Boards to include, beyond their board membership, a broad range of stakeholders in their work and to ensure that the community was actively involved in their work. The need to involve local healthwatch (see Chapter 5) and the voluntary and community sector (see Chapter 6) in JSNAs and JHWSs, especially in engaging with and communicating the views of the public and of people in vulnerable circumstances, was heavily emphasized. As already noted, the guidance urged county council Health and Wellbeing Boards to work closely with district councils. Guidance was also provided on other matters relating to the work of Health and Wellbeing Boards, such as promoting service integration and pharmaceutical needs assessments (DH, 2013a).

The development of shadow Health and Wellbeing Boards was analysed by the King's Fund (Humphries et al., 2012). This found that Health and Wellbeing Boards attracted wide support and offered opportunities to join up services and create new partnerships, while potentially creating greater democratic accountability. The report was based on a survey of 50 local authorities and an in-depth analysis of two local authority areas. It found that some Health and Wellbeing Boards had been innovative in engaging with stakeholders, including the public and voluntary sector. Health and Wellbeing Boards were seen as strengthening engagement with CCGs, but as less effective in engaging with secondary healthcare providers. The research found that Health and Wellbeing Boards needed to be clear about what they could achieve. Potential tensions were identified between some of their functions, notably overseeing commissioning and promoting integration, and they needed to be able to deal with these. There was also some uncertainty about the ability of boards to influence the NHS Commissioning Board (now NHS England) to develop local priorities (as opposed to national policy imperatives), and about the responsibilities of the new NHS bodies. This issue was picked up subsequently by the Conmmunities and Local Government Committee (2013), which observed that while NHS England should have regard to JSNAs and JHWSs, in practice the accountability mechanisms were weak.

The King's Fund study further argued that a stronger national framework would be needed to integrate care. The biggest challenge identified for Health and Wellbeing Boards was the need to deliver strong, credible and shared leadership across local organizational boundaries in a period of severe financial restraint. The discretion given to local authorities in establishing Health and Wellbeing Boards was responsible for a considerable variation in approach. This was not regarded as necessarily a bad thing provided that lessons could be learned from these diverse experiences.

Another study (Kuznetsova, 2012) also found a high level of support for Health and Wellbeing Boards among councils and shadow board members. This report identified great opportunities to improve health and to increase community participation in health. But it also found a number of potential problems, including territorialism and organizational divisions. It argued that strong leadership would be needed to mobilize actors across different organizations and departments (see also Communities and Local Government Committee, 2013). Particular problems of joint working were identified in two-tier authorities (see above). The report also called for more powers, duties and incentives to ensure that organizations worked together for the benefit of public health and well-being. Its recommendations included: a duty on all public bodies to cooperate with the JHWS; powers for Health and Wellbeing Board chairs to call in local authority departments to ensure that service commissioning and delivery took the JHWS into account; cross-representation on Health and Wellbeing Boards between neighbouring areas; greater scrutiny of Health and Wellbeing Boards by district councils in two-tier areas; establishment of provider panels to link to the design and implementation of the JHWS; and powers for Health and Wellbeing Boards to challenge decisions by the NHS Commissioning Board (NHS England) where these could be demonstrated to have an adverse effect. The report also recommended that Health and Wellbeing Boards should publish a public involvement strategy. Other recommendations included piloting of pooled budget arrangements to identify potential barriers, and explicit agreements to demonstrate the commitment and contribution of individual board members.

The establishment of Health and Wellbeing Boards in shadow form has contributed a great deal to our understanding of what is likely to be achieved now they are statutory bodies. It also gives us an insight into their working practices and their limitations (see Churchill, 2012; NHS Confederation et al., 2012a, 2012b, 2012c, 2012d). Some local areas have already used their Health and Wellbeing Boards to set clear objectives and priorities, to experiment with new ways of service provision, and to promote service integration. They have also begun to use Health and Wellbeing Boards to challenge health inequalities. However, it is acknowledged that the powers of Health and Wellbeing Boards, although stronger than originally proposed, are weaker than they might have been. A veto power on commissioning plans would have given Health and Wellbeing Boards much more bite. The new bodies also lack budgetary and financial powers. This is widely acknowledged. Indeed, it is recognized that Health and Wellbeing Boards will have to focus more on 'soft power', strengthening cooperation by building relationships and changing the culture of local health and social care bodies (Communities and Local Government Committee, 2013). It remains to be seen how successful they will be in this regard and whether or not their institutional framework and powers will need to be revised and strengthened to enable them to fulfil their important role.

Building partnerships through multidisciplinary and interprofessional working

Another important area of partnership highlighted by the Coalition, and by previous governments too, was multidisciplinary and interprofessional working in public health. Throughout the history of public health, conflict between different professions has been evident. During the twentieth century, for example, interprofessional conflicts occurred between GPs and public health doctors, between GPs and nurses, midwives and health visitors, and public health medicine and non-medical public health practitioners (Lewis, 1986). Even when overt conflict was absent, there was often suspicion between different professional groups, linked primarily to battles over status and territory. There were attempts to control aspects of public health and limit the role of others who could contribute. This led to fragmentation, a weakening of public health in relation to clinical medicine, and the exclusion and marginalization of professionals, workers and holders of other forms of knowledge and expertise (such as in the areas of community development, environmental health and housing, for example) from mainstream public health practice.

Reforms to the structure of the NHS and local government had a limited impact on these problems. It has long been acknowledged that simply changing organizational structures does not necessarily produce greater interprofessional cooperation (Ottewill and Wall, 1990; Audit Scotland, 2011). Indeed, it can make things worse. For example, removing the public health function from local government in 1974 and transferring it to the NHS served only to further marginalize its practitioners. In the late 1980s, government sought to restore their status with the Acheson reforms, establishing DPHs at local level and renaming community medicine specialists as consultants in public health medicine. Meanwhile, there were moves to give non-medical practitioners greater status, with the Faculty of Public Health Medicine opening its doors to non-medics in the late 1990s, and in 2003 symbolically changing its name to the Faculty of Public Health. The Labour Government's White Paper, *Saving Lives* (Cm 4386, 1999) attempted to break down barriers further by establishing the principle that non-medical public health professionals could become specialists with equivalent status to consultants in public health medicine. In 2002, non-medics were able to become DPHs. However, as Hunter et al. (2007) noted, medical hegemony remained. Non-medical DPHs remained in a minority and were paid less than those who were medically qualified (Naidoo et al., 2003). Furthermore, doctors retained a strong influence over professional accreditation, training and standards in this field (Evans, 2003). Over 10 years after this initiative was introduced, around a quarter of senior public health professionals are not medically qualified (Jacques, 2013).

Sir Liam Donaldson, as Chief Medical Officer, had earlier signalled that all elements of the public health workforce must be acknowledged (DH, 2001). He identified three broad categories within the public health workforce: public health consultants and specialists working at a senior level of management or with a high level of expertise (for example, DPHs and consultants in public health medicine); professionals spending a major part of their time in public health practice (for example, health visitors and environmental health officers); and professionals with a contribution to make to public health but who may not recognize this (for example, teachers, social workers, housing officers and some healthcare professionals). The Donaldson Report stated that the contribution of the wider public health workforce must be acknowledged, and envisaged that future leadership of public health would come from a wider range of professional backgrounds. It maintained that progress must be made on making public health more multidisciplinary. The report also called for the strengthening of public health networks (see below and Chapter 3), national workforce targets and development plans, and core competences for public health specialists and standards of accreditation.

The subsequent White Paper, *Choosing Health* (Cm 6374, 2004), reiterated the importance of workforce planning, skills development and interprofessional and multidisciplinary working. Public health networks were encouraged to pool resources and build capacity, as well as bring together different public health professions and workers. Even so, the medical profession remained powerful within these networks and in the multidisciplinary and multiprofessional teams in the NHS. Evidence remained of the marginalization and exclusion of professional groups and workers who could contribute greatly to public health practice and policy (Mallinson et al., 2006; Hunter et al., 2007; Wills and Ellison, 2007). Team-working and fragmentation remained problematic (Evans, 2003; Chapman et al., 2005). Problems of underresourcing the public health function, skill shortages and poor morale among the public health workforce continued

(Chapman et al., 2005; Hunter et al., 2007; Wanless, 2007; Faculty of Public Health, 2008). The number of public health specialists and other key professional groups vital to public health – notably school nurses, health visitors and health promotion specialists – fell (Ball and Pike, 2005; Derrett and Burke, 2006; Audit Commission, 2010b). Attempts were made to reiterate the importance of these groups (see Griffiths and Dark, 2006), but despite the commitment to strengthen public health workforce planning, not just in the NHS but across local government and the voluntary sector, there was little progress. On a more positive note, a skills and career framework in public health, complementing national occupational standards, was introduced. This provided a basis on which to develop a multidisciplinary and multiprofessional workforce. However, without the necessary resources and long-term strategic planning at national and local level, it was doubtful that much progress would be made.

Towards the end of Labour's period in office, public health workforce planning once again returned the agenda (DH, 2008; NHS Workforce Review Team, 2009). However, the task of following this through fell to the Coalition government. As noted, the Coalition embarked on radical reforms, with wide-ranging implications for the public health workforce. These included the transfer of key public health responsibilities to local government, the establishment of a national public health service in the form of Public Health England, the abolition of PCTs and SHAs, and the transfer of local health service commissioning to CCGs. Some of these changes had potential for greater integration of the public health workforce. For example, the location of key public health functions in local government raised the prospect of bringing public health specialists and practitioners into closer contact with the wider workforce – such as those working in housing, planning, education, social services and transport. Meanwhile, Public Health England offered an opportunity to bring different forms of professional expertise together at national level and facilitate strategic planning of the public health workforce. Clinical commissioning, particularly in the context of Health and Wellbeing Boards, JSNAs and JHWSs, could provide an opportunity to integrate the work of different professions and workers to support the promotion of health and well-being. However, none of this was guaranteed and, indeed, there was criticism that the reforms would fragment public health services and by implication the workforce that provided them. A further concern was that reorganization was itself damaging and would disrupt existing relationships between professionals at local level.

The government sought to reassure critics by amending the composition of CCGs (as discussed above) and by agreeing to multiprofessional advisory structures in the commissioning process that included public health expertise. It also consulted on a workforce strategy for the public health system (DH, 2012c). This ran alongside plans to ensure a smooth transition of staff to the new public health structures. The public health workforce consultation document reflected the reforms to the NHS mentioned earlier. It also took into account changes to the system of funding and commissioning education and training for the health workforce (see DH, 2010b). This involved the creation of Local Education and Training Boards (LETBs), partnership bodies that would develop local strategies and allocate resources. LETBs would be authorized and funded by a national body, Health Education England, that would monitor their performance against an outcomes framework.

The public health workforce strategy was finalized in 2013 (DH, Public Health England and LGA, 2013) This set out a vision that the public health workforce would be known for its expertise, professionalism, commitment to population health and well-being, and flexibility, especially with regard to working in partnership across organizational boundaries. Key themes of this strategy were: capacity-building; the improvement of career pathways; strengthening the contribution of nurses and midwives to public health; the maintenance of high standards of professional conduct; improvements in data related to the public health workforce; and clearer responsibilities for workforce development. Specific actions promised included: the use of an existing review of the public health skills and career framework to refine the relevance of this framework for local authorities and develop a new skills 'passport' for public health; the development of leadership programmes; efforts (involving Public Health England, the Department of Health, the Nursing and Midwifery Council and others) to support and develop the public health nursing and midwifery contribution to population health and the public health outcomes framework; the development of a knowledge and information workforce; development of the non-medical scientific workforce; measures to strengthen academic public health and strengthen links between academia and practitioners; and the establishment of a minimum dataset for the public health workforce to support workforce planning. In addition, Health Education England was given the task of leading on workforce planning, education and training, with advice and support from Public Health England; it was proposed that a lead LETB for public health be identified; and the Faculty of Public Health was tasked with updating and developing the specialist public health curriculum and assessment systems. The strategy reiterated an earlier commitment that statutory regulation would be extended to non-medical public health specialists. Finally, further advice and guidance was promised on ideas for local innovation in workforce development and the alignment of skills with local community priorities, the development of which was to be led by the Local Government Association.

The above discussion relates to England, but it should be noted that other parts of the UK have faced similar problems with regard to their public health workforces and have sought to address them. In Wales, for example, a national workforce development plan for public health was developed (Public Health Wales, 2011). This called for a more coordinated approach to workforce development, emphasized the need to involve the wider public health workforce, and underlined the importance of the monitoring and evaluation of initiatives. The national public health body, Public Health Wales, was given the task of leading the strategy. Specific priorities identified included: establishing a network of learning and development contacts across health boards, local government and the voluntary sector; developing an introductory-level course on core public health skills that would be available to professionals contributing to public health; developing career pathways; and working with further and higher education institutions to respond to gaps in training needs.

Conclusion

The Cameron government's radical reforms of the NHS and the public health system had wide implications for partnership working. On the one hand, they promised improvements through the inclusiveness of Health and Wellbeing Boards, requirements to produce JSNAs/JHWSs and obligations on commissioning bodies to have regard to them, the leadership role of Public Health England, and the relocation of key public health functions and personnel to local government. On the other hand, there were doubts that these would be achieved and indeed that existing arrangements and relationships would be undermined. The extensive nature of the reforms, the abolition of some institutions (PCTs and SHAs) and the creation of new bodies (Public Health England, CCGs and NHS England) meant that it would take time to implement the changes and re-establish working relationships and partnerships. This was exacerbated by differences in organizational boundaries at local level between the various NHS organizations and local authorities. Furthermore, there was concern that some of the reforms would cause a deterioration in partnership working through further fragmentation, overlap and duplication of public health functions. There was also disquiet about the narrow agenda of CCGs and their ability to sidestep public health responsibilities, notwithstanding efforts to prevent them from doing so. Furthermore, while Health and Wellbeing Boards were widely welcomed, most observers agreed that they lacked formal powers and that at some stage this would probably have to be revisited. In essence, the Coalition's reforms were very much a leap in the dark, and it will be some time before it becomes clear whether the quality of partnership working in public health had improved, deteriorated or stayed the same.

There was also concern that the Coalition had dismantled structures and processes established by the previous government that had provided useful foundations for partnership working in public health, notably LAAs and CAAs. The abolition of regional structures, notably GORs, SHAs and the regional public health observatories (now part of Public Health England), was also seen in some quarters as damaging to collaboration. Against this, however, it must be noted that some initiatives were developed further (notably JSNAs and 'place-based' initiatives such as Whole-Place and community budgets). Moreover, the Coalition continued to emphasize the importance of partnership and collaboration to tackle key issues such as obesity, alcohol misuse and health inequalities. Its commitment, however, was undermined in the eyes of many public health leaders by the decision to scrap its public health Cabinet committee in November 2012 (Campbell, 2012). From their perspective, this committee – heralded as a key coordinating mechanism in the *Healthy Lives, Healthy People* White Paper (Cm 7985, 2010) – was an important symbol of government leadership on public health and cross-departmental commitment on tackling preventable causes of illness.

Notably, a further report from the NHS Future Forum (2012) also made it clear that the government should do more to ensure that the whole health system could do more to prevent poor health. In particular, it wanted health service providers to be given clearer responsibilities for the prevention of ill health and the promotion of healthy living, building these into their everyday business and making every contact with patients count. The report's recommendations included a strategy for improving the health and well-being of health service staff, improvements in staff training, sharing of information and best practice, and better incentives and performance frameworks to incentivize health service organizations and professionals to promote health and prevent illness. The report also identified partnerships – within the NHS, and between health service organizations and other local service providers – as being crucial to improving health and well-being.

5 Partnerships with the community and citizens

Introduction

An increasingly important dimension of partnership working is engagement with communities and citizens. This chapter explores this aspect of partnerships in some detail. It begins by analysing community participation as a basis for partnership and its potential to address public health challenges. Policy initiatives to extend and improve community participation and partnership are then examined, including reforms of the public involvement system in the NHS, other relevant participation initiatives and community development approaches. The primary focus again is upon England, although the experiences of Scotland, Wales and Northern Ireland are also examined (see Box 5.3).

Community participation

Terminology and frameworks

One of the main problems faced when analysing community participation is that the terminology is imprecise and contested. At a very simple level, community participation means involving people in decisions and actions that affect their welfare. However, difficulties arise when moving beyond this. These stem from the contested nature of both 'community' and 'participation'. The term 'community' is often used imprecisely (Taylor, 2003). It is frequently deployed as a rhetorical device to conjure up the notion of a closely knit and supportive social framework (Baum, 2002), even though society is actually fragmented into groups, networks and interests (Gilchrist, 2006). Moreover, the term does not accurately capture the variety of roles played by individual citizens and groups in their interactions with state agencies.

In the health arena, there is reference to community, public and citizen participation as well as participation on the part of health consumers, lay people, patients, carers, service users, advocates (and even 'survivors'). Although, somewhat confusingly, such terms are often used interchangeably, each is distinctive and some are highly contested (Wait and Nolte, 2006). For example, some argue that 'health consumer' implies a market-oriented ethos that structures relationships between people and public services in an inappropriate way (Long, 1999). Others, meanwhile, have devised hybrid terms, such as 'citizen-consumers' to capture new constructions that place greater emphasis on choice and consumerism but that also draw on collective notions of citizenship (Clarke et al., 2007).

Similarly, there is disagreement over the meaning of 'participation'. Again, the situation is exacerbated by the use of different terms interchangeably, such as 'consultation', 'involvement', 'empowerment' and 'engagement', even though these have different meanings (Wait and Nolte, 2006). There has long been a distinction, for example, between empowerment, which implies that people have a high degree of control and self-determination (Laverack, 2005), and involvement or engagement, where people have a voice, and maybe have some influence over policy and services, but within a framework controlled by the authorities, and consultation, in which people have an even more passive role. Some have attempted to clarify this terminology by identifying degrees of participation. Perhaps the best known is 'Arnstein's ladder' of citizen participation (Arnstein, 1969). This identifies a hierarchy of activities, those at the top end yielding more power to the citizen (citizen control, power and partnership) compared with those which cede less power (placation, consultation, information), and those at the bottom where the citizen is in an even weaker position (therapy, manipulation) (see also Feingold, 1977; Baum, 2002). In contrast, Davidson (1998), rejecting a hierarchical approach, formulated a 'wheel of participation', with four different categories of participation – information, consultation, participation and empowerment – having equal value, some being more appropriate in certain situations than others.

Others have proposed more complex frameworks, arguing that these capture the evolutionary and dynamic nature of participation and the diversity of citizens and their various roles and contexts. Fung (2006) formulated a 'participation cube' reflecting three dimensions along which degrees of participation could be represented: participant selection (ranging from inclusive to exclusive selection criteria and mechanisms); communication and decision-making (ranging from active forms of participation such as contributing expertise to passive forms such as listening); and authority and power (ranging from control by participants through to various degrees of dependence on authority). In similar vein, Charles and De Maio (1993) conceptualized public participation in healthcare as three-dimensional (Figure 5.1). The first dimension of their model, reflecting Arnstein, relates to degrees of citizen control (consultation, partnership and lay domination). The second refers to domains of participatory activity (macro-level policy, service design and individual treatment), while the third reflects the different role perspectives (the narrower user perspective and the wider public policy perspective).

Tritter and McCallum (2006) also propose an alternative analogy to the simple hierarchy of Arnstein's ladder, which, they argue, fails to capture the dynamic and evolutionary nature of user involvement and does not account for the 'agency' of users themselves, who may actively choose different methods of involvement in relation to different issues at different times (and may of course wish not to be involved at all). Instead of a 'ladder', Tritter and McCallum propose a 'mosaic' in which a picture is created that is the product of a complex and dynamic relationship between many different tiles (representing the spatial interactions between users, communities, voluntary organizations and the healthcare system).

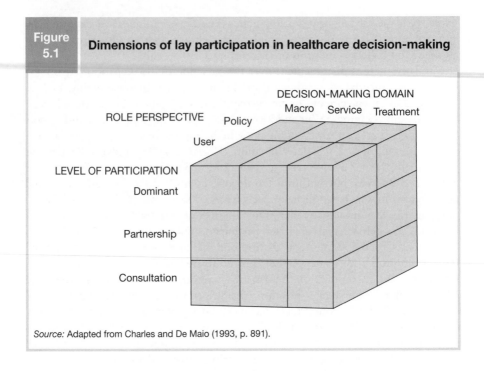

Figure 5.1 Dimensions of lay participation in healthcare decision-making

Source: Adapted from Charles and De Maio (1993, p. 891).

Participation roles and practices

Research into participation in health has found that it incorporates many roles and relationships and is often context-specific. Litva et al. (2009) examined the experiences in the field of clinical governance of lay people drawn from different groups (citizens, patient user groups, health interest groups and frequent service users) and found that people adopted different 'role perspectives' (citizen, advocate and consumer). Furthermore, these groups varied according to their preferred mode of participation (which included 'overseeing' practices such as performance management, providing and receiving information about activities, and working in partnership with clinicians). Moreover, these preferences varied according to the different aspects of clinical governance under consideration (improving and assessing services, dealing with poor performance, and education/training).

Others have also observed that community participation involves lay people undertaking different functions, some of which conflict. Martin (2008) found that there are democratic (or representative) and technocratic tendencies in lay participation and that these can pull in different directions. While an emphasis on representation tends to broaden lay participation (in order that different social groups are represented), the focus on the technical expertise of service users tends to narrow it. This does not necessarily mean that it is impossible to involve lay people effectively in decision-making. But it does raise questions about how this can be done in order to satisfy different criteria for 'representation' and 'expertise', while at the same time avoiding the incorporation, capture and professionalization of lay participation, which undermines its fundamental ethos (see Learmonth et al., 2009). Participation need not, however, always involve lay people within institutional structures. Bang (2005) distinguished 'expert citizens' (those who seek to represent views within recognized systems of representation such as voluntary organizations and policy networks) from 'everyday makers' ('doers' who prefer to engage in concrete activities leading to their desired ends rather than articulate the views of others). The latter can be influential, even if they do not participate in a conventional manner (they could, for example, establish a self-help group or become a volunteer).

There is much scepticism that institutional structures actually further the empowerment of citizens. Blaug (2002) identifies two types of democracy. *Incumbent democracy* is institutional and representative, and in line with elite norms. It seeks to preserve existing institutions by maximizing orderly participation, and is controlled and stable. *Critical democracy*, however, is more deliberative and challenges existing norms. It is potentially more empowering and personal, and involves direct participation on the part of citizens. Blaug's first type of democracy is akin to Eriksson's (2012) concept of a 'self-service society', in which participation is restricted to technical issues of service provision. This places additional responsibilities on citizens, emphasizes their role as consumers, and limits the scope of political debate. Meanwhile, Barnes et al. (2007) have categorized different public participation discourses reflecting various roles and activities undertaken by citizens and the reasons for involving them. Hence citizens can be seen as 'empowered' (reflecting a desire to give them power), 'consuming' (giving them choices), 'stakeholding' (giving them a voice and a stake in governance) and 'responsible' (having obligations and duties, taking responsibility for themselves and being active citizens).

Different concepts of participation reflect not only the complex governance roles of citizens and communities, but also the strategies of the state in seeking to maintain its power and capacity to govern. For Blaug, efforts to engineer democracy through the 'top-down' approaches of incumbent democracy will ultimately fail. Indeed, their underlying purpose is to preserve existing institutions and elites. This is not to say, however, that government and public bodies are necessarily ill-intentioned. Indeed, some genuinely see themselves as champions of participation and empowerment. However, as Blaug, suggested, such noble aims founder, and it is often the case that 'those genuinely seeking to increase participation only discover their ambivalence toward popular input at the point where their own power is directly threatened' (Blaug, 2002, p. 109). Although Barnes et al. (2007) identified similar limits to citizen participation, they acknowledged that participation may create opportunities and spaces that enable new and challenging ideas to develop, potentially leading to greater empowerment. Martin (2008) agreed, highlighting for example the important mediating role of lay people in NHS public involvement structures and their potential to contribute to citizen governance through their knowledge of the community. Also relevant here is Learmonth et al. (2009), who argued that local patient and public involvement bodies should be given space and time to pursue their own agenda, to enable them to challenge authoritative decisions and encourage open public debates about health and health services.

Why encourage community participation and partnership in public health?

Community participation in public health has been based on two main arguments (Barnes et al., 2007; Coulter, 2009; Heritage and Dooris, 2009). The first is that participation will improve the accountability and responsiveness of policy-makers to the public and strengthen the legitimacy of their policies (Cooper et al., 1995; Barnes et al., 2007). Second, public health policies and services will become more effective as a result of this. Greater participation might lead to the identification of important issues that might otherwise be ignored or neglected. Participation may improve the identification of needs, identify obstacles to potentially effective initiatives, and bring in new ideas about policy and service provision. It may also improve implementation by strengthening capacity, mobilizing community resources, promoting cohesion, enabling communities to have ownership of initiatives, contributing to community development, and building social capital (Box 5.1; DH, 2001; Barnes et al., 2007; Strategic Review of Health Inequalities in England, 2010).

Box 5.1	Social capital

Social capital is the benefit derived from participation in social relationships (Putnam, 2000; Johnston and Percy Smith, 2003). Putnam (1993, pp. 35–6) defines it as 'features of social organizations, such as networks, norms and trust, that facilitate action and cooperation for mutual benefit.' However, the concept has been contested, and its benefits challenged. For example, some forms of social capital, which strengthen the solidarity of subgroups within society, appear to fragment rather than strengthen social cohesion (Portes, 1998; Haynes, 2009). Nonetheless, with regard to health, a number of potential benefits are linked to social capital (Kawachi and Berkman, 2003; Borgonovi, 2010). Social capital may increase the dissemination of information about healthy lifestyles and facilitate their adoption; it can strengthen psychosocial support and thereby improve well-being and reduce stress-related illness; and it may strengthen community solidarity and underpin community action to campaign for measures that improve health and well-being. A number of empirical studies have found that individuals and communities with higher levels of social capital tend to have better health (Kaplan et al., 1996; McCulloch, 2001; Veenstra et al., 2005; Li, 2007; Freidli, 2009; Borgonovi, 2010), although others are more sceptical (Cattell, 2001; Muntaner et al., 2001; Almedom, 2005).

It is widely believed that health and well-being can be improved by encouraging people and communities to participate (Wanless, 2004; Naidoo and Wills, 2005). Participation may lead to people taking greater responsibility for their own health, developing their own initiatives as well as contributing to the development of public policies. 'Co-production' may expand, as the service users, the public, and voluntary and community organizations work jointly with public authorities to improve services and policy outcomes (Boyle and Harris, 2009). Participation may enable lay knowledge and experiences to be incorporated into public policies, public service delivery and voluntary initiatives, leading to policy and service innovation. Empowerment may directly lead to positive changes in people's health and well-being (Laverack, 2005) by strengthening self-esteem and confidence among participants while helping to tackle social exclusion and inequity by reaching out to those not normally included in decision-making or who face obstacles in making their voices heard (Strategic Review of Health Inequalities in England, 2010). The involvement of lay people in service delivery (as volunteers or community champions) may be justified on several grounds. It may reduce barriers between service providers and communities, particularly those who are disadvantaged, improve communication, increase service capacity, give opportunities for skills development, training and employment, provide peer support for those wishing to improve their health, and act as a two-way conduit for the transmission of health promotion messages through social networks and the communication of community knowledge to decision-makers (South et al., 2010, 2012).

Policies on community participation and partnerships in health

Political support for community participation

The belief that improvements in public health and well-being require active participation is reflected in policies at all levels of health governance. Community participation was identified as a key element in the World Health Organization (WHO) Health for All strategy (WHO, 1981, 1998a; WHO Regional Office for Europe, 1999a), in declarations and charters on health promotion (WHO and UNICEF, 1978; WHO, 1986, 1997), and in specific programmes (such as Healthy Cities; see Heritage and Dooris, 2009). The role of communities and voluntary organizations has been emphasized in global strategies in relation to specific problems, such as obesity and alcohol (see WHO, 2004, 2010b). Participation and partnership in health is also an important theme in European public policy, reflected in documents published by the Council of Europe (2000); European Union (EU; Commission of the European Communities, 2007) and the WHO Regional Office for Europe (2011).

Since the late 1990s, government policies in England have explicitly referred to community involvement in public health. *Saving Lives* (Cm 4386, 1999) commented on the importance of involving people as active participants in their own health and that of their communities. *Choosing Health* echoed this, stating that 'Communities are vital in improving health and can play a significant role in promoting individual self-esteem and mental well-being and reducing exclusion' (Cm 6374, 2004, p. 79). Subsequently, *Our Health, Our Care, Our Say* proposed a greater voice for the public and individual services users, especially in the commissioning of health and social care services (Cm 6737, 2006). Notably, community participation was encouraged in related policy areas, such as environmental sustainability (Rask et al., 2011), parenting and child well-being (for example, Sure Start and related initiatives; see Box 3.2) and economic and social regeneration (Cm 4911, 2000; ODPM, 2003). More generally, New Labour's public service reforms created pressures to incorporate service user, public and community perspectives, leading to the reform of participation structures and systems (Clarke and Newman, 1997; Cm 6939, 2006; Clarke et al., 2007; Cm 7427, 2008; Newman and Clarke, 2009).

Subsequently, the Conservative Party leader David Cameron championed the 'Big Society', and this has since become a prominent theme of the Coalition's policy. The concept is vague and ambiguous, but essentially implies a shift in power and responsibility from the state to civil society, voluntary organizations and individuals (Box 5.2). This underlying principle is linked to policies that claim to decentralize power, make available information to the public (for instance, on social problems and public services) and provide financial support for voluntary activities (through a 'Big Society Bank' and other funding streams). In relation to health, three areas of action have been identified: social action, public service reforms and community empowerment (Taylor et al., 2011). More specifically, policies on public health have emphasized the role of community engagement and the inclusion of voluntary and community organizations as partners in securing health improvements and providing public health services (Cm 7881, 2010; Cm 7985, 2010).

Box 5.2	The Big Society

David Cameron, the leader of the Conservative Party and subsequently Prime Minister in the Conservative–Liberal Democrat Coalition government, set out his vision of the 'Big Society' before and after the General Election of 2010. The basic idea was to restructure the relationship between the state and society by shifting power and responsibility from the former to the latter (Pattie and Johnston, 2011). The Cameron government set out the main dimensions of this programme as follows (Cabinet Office, 2010):

- To give communities more powers.
- To encourage people to take an active role in their communities.
- To transfer power from central to local government.
- To support cooperatives, mutuals, charities and social enterprises, and especially to help them run public services.
- To publish government information about social problems and public services.

The Big Society was a rhetorical device to reposition the Conservative Party as a centre-right party, acknowledging the importance of communities and civil society (Corbett and Walker, 2012). This enabled Cameron to distance himself and his party from the neoliberal Conservative governments of the 1980s and 1990s (notably that of Margaret Thatcher, who famously commented that 'there is no such thing as society'). An emphasis on social action and community empowerment also enabled Cameron to criticize the 'Big Government' approach he associated with previous Labour governments. In fact, the picture is more complex than this. As Davies (2012) points out, even Thatcherism had a notion of community and acknowledged the importance of active citizenship in relation to both the market economy and social welfare. Furthermore, although New Labour presided over a considerable growth in central government, it adopted a similar rhetoric of decentralization, pluralism in the supply of public services, public information about services, local autonomy, community empowerment and active citizenship.

As the Select Committee on Public Administration (2011, p. 9) stated: 'The Big Society is not a new concept. It builds on a wealth of traditions and ideas about strengthening communities, civic action and co-ownership of public services.' Cameron's Big Society resonated with ideas of previous Conservative thinkers, such as Edmund Burke's affection for the 'little platoon we belong to in society' (Burke, 1987). But it was not an exclusively Conservative idea. Concepts of mutualism and social solidarity are embedded in socialist thought (notably the cooperative movement, trade unionism and, more recently, communitarianism). The Big Society echoes cultural traditions that cut across ideological and party political lines, recalling the great historian A.J.P. Taylor's 'great army of busybodies' sustaining the public life of England (cited in Hilton and McKay, 2011, p. 47).

Cameron drew on recent Conservative thinkers who had attempted to reformulate modern Conservativism, rejecting the 'free market' and individualism and placing greater emphasis on active citizenship, community empowerment, building social capital and trust, while addressing poverty, disadvantage and inequality (see, for example, Blond, 2010; Norman, 2010). However, despite attempts to bolster its intellectual underpinnings, the Big Society is poorly understood by government and the general public (ACEVO, 2010; Hudson, 2011; Select Committee on Public Administration, 2011, 2012). Moreover, there is a danger that 'Big Society' policies are based upon false premises. Key assumptions have been criticized, for example that the voluntary sector can easily take on complex roles currently carried out by the state (see Chapter 6), or that deep-rooted social and economic problems can be easily resolved at a local level. Indeed, one of the misapprehensions of adherents of the Big Society is that the state and the voluntary sector are part of a zero-sum game – an advance in one sector leads to a recession of the other – which has historically not been the case (Hilton and McKay, 2011).

In addition, practical problems have plagued the Big Society initiative. The policy had a number of 'false starts' and drifted somewhat. The resignation in May 2011 of a key advisor (Lord Wei), less than a year after he had been appointed, was embarrassing for the government. The coherence of policies across Whitehall has been questioned, amid calls for clearer leadership (ACEVO, 2011; Select Committee on Public Administration, 2011). There are suspicions that the policy is merely a cover for policies to subject public services to market forces and privatize them, while reducing public expenditure (Hudson, 2011; Corbett and Walker, 2012). Paradoxically, as Pattie and Johnston (2011, p. 420) have observed, 'fiscal retrenchment may yet prove the Big Society's Achilles' heel'. The voluntary sector, which is seen as vital to the achievement of the Big Society, has faced substantial cuts in public funding, placing the project in some jeopardy (see Chapter 6). There are also fears that the vitality and autonomy of this sector may be lost if it takes on a greater role in public service delivery. Another danger is that, by taking on public services in an era of austerity, voluntary organizations could be identified as conspirators in budget cuts and service reduction, undermining public trust in them. Other problems include deficits in volunteering (Pattie and Johnston, 2011), and more is needed to enable people to take on such responsibilities within their busy lives (NEF, 2010; ACEVO, 2011). A further problem is that not all local areas or policy sectors have the same level of social capacity and resources (NEF, 2010; ACEVO, 2011; Pattie and Johnston, 2011). Unless ways are found of addressing this, a greater reliance on the Big Society could widen rather than reduce social inequalities and undermine social cohesion.

Social trends, evidence and principles

Recent social trends have promoted community participation in health (Williamson, 1992; Laverack, 2005), including greater health literacy, the expansion of information about health (especially through the Internet), the growth in media coverage of health issues, health consumerism and the greater value placed on lay experiences of health and illness. There has also been a growth in active citizenship, reflected in health social movements and the voluntary health sector (discussed in Chapter 6).

However, despite the support for promoting community participation, there is a dearth of hard evidence on how it actually contributes to health improvement (Select Committee on Public Administration, 2008a). Reviews of the impact of participation in the health field show that the main focus of research is on health services rather than public health (Daykin et al., 2007). Research into community participation in public health has been criticized for its poor quality and an inability to demonstrate clear and direct outcomes from interventions. This is largely a problem of study design, given the difficulties of capturing the health impact of interventions that seek to increase community and individual participation. More transparent, systematic and robustly designed research may help (Craig et al., 2008; NICE, 2008c; Bonell, C. et al., 2011; Cousens et al., 2011). Nonetheless, the limited evidence available provides some justification for pursuing strategies and programmes in this area (see Woodall et al., 2010). Participation strategies can improve confidence and self-esteem, promote a greater sense of personal control, increase knowledge, awareness and skills and possibly behavioural change, improve health status (and disease management when focused on people with long-term conditions), and promote a greater sense of community and stronger social networks, thereby contributing to social capital.

There is evidence on the practice of community participation in health, which has enabled the development of principles of good practice (see NICE, 2008c; Coulter, 2009). Others too have identified general principles that identify circumstances and practices in which public participation can be beneficial (and conversely where it might not be effective), and these can also be applied to health and wellbeing (Irvine and Stansbury, 2004; NCC and Involve, 2008; Select Committee on Public Administration, 2008a). The main conclusions of this work are that participation should be carried out for clear and genuine reasons rather than tokenism, must be transparent and have integrity, must address barriers that prevent people in general and specific groups from participating, must not overburden people or cause undue delays in decision-making, must be properly resourced, work to a realistic timetable and work with the community and its networks and organizations, must be based on previous evidence about what is effective and be properly evaluated, and must have an impact that is clearly communicated to participants.

Community participation in the NHS

This section explores initiatives to introduce and strengthen community participation specifically in relation to health (and, more recently, social care) services. Although the main focus of these efforts has been upon diagnostic, treatment and care services, they have had important implications for public health. Some health (and social care) services have an important prevention or health promotion dimension to their work. Moreover, health and social care planning has increasingly involved assessments of the population's health needs and priorities, which is a key public health function.

From the inception of the NHS, lay people have been appointed to health boards and authorities. In the 1970s, policy-makers acknowledged that public accountability of health services had to be strengthened. In 1974, Community Health Councils (CHCs) were established as the patients' watchdog for the NHS in England and Wales, with similar bodies established in Northern Ireland and Scotland (Gerrard, 2006; Hogg, 2009). CHCs were statutory bodies established in each district, their members chosen by voluntary organizations, local authorities and NHS regions, and they employed a small number of staff. They were funded by the NHS regions (giving them greater independence than if they had been funded by the local NHS bodies they were holding to account). CHCs were required to produce an annual report and given a statutory right of consultation on local health service reorganizations. They undertook a number of other roles: monitoring local health services and suggesting improvements, obtaining and providing information about services, and assistance with complaints. Encouraged by government, many CHCs developed a public health role, which included undertaking health surveys, participating in health promotion campaigns, providing information about health and monitoring health education services.

However, CHCs had limited financial and staffing resources, and few statutory powers. Although they varied considerably in their activities, reflecting to some extent differences in local needs and contexts, there was a lack of consistency in standards. A national body, the Association of Community Health Councils for England and Wales (ACHCEW), was established to lead and represent the sector, but this proved difficult. There was also a problem of democratic legitimacy, although some CHCs made great efforts to work with and involve their communities. In the 1980s and 1990s, NHS bodies began to bypass CHCs, using alternative techniques for gauging public opinion and legitimizing their policies (such as surveys, focus groups, patients' forums, consultation exercises and citizens' juries). The advent of the internal market in the 1990s created a stronger momentum for the uptake of these techniques, and the NHS was urged to listen to the views of patients, users and carers when planning and commissioning services. Subsequently in 1996, a Patient Partnership Strategy was devised to promote greater user choice and involvement (NHS Executive, 1996). Although this focused on individual patient involvement, it was acknowledged that the NHS bodies should seek to consult and involve both the public and service users collectively through voluntary organizations. They were also encouraged to involve people in public health issues, to identify priorities for action and to strengthen community development approaches in health (see below).

Patient and public involvement under New Labour

Efforts to extend patient and public involvement developed in an unsystematic way and were criticized for being fragmented (NHS Executive et al., 1998). The

New Labour government then abolished CHCs and the ACHCEW, replacing them with a new system, consisting of the following (DH, 1999; Cm 4818, 2000):

- Patient Advice and Liaison Services (PALS) based in Primary Care Trusts (PCTs) and NHS Trusts, giving advice and information to patients, relatives and carers, and helping to resolve problems at an early stage.
- Independent Complaints Advocacy Services (ICAS), funded by government but provided by voluntary organizations to assist and support people wishing to make a complaint about NHS-funded services.
- Patient and Public Involvement Forums (PPIFs) in each PCT and NHS Trust, advising them on the views of patients, users, carers and the wider public, and monitoring the quality of local services.
- Health Overview and Scrutiny Committees (HOSCs), based in local authorities, monitoring and reviewing local health issues and health services and being consulted when substantial service changes are proposed (see Chapter 3).
- A new national statutory body, the Commission for Patient and Public Involvement in Health (CPPIH), promoting patient and public involvement, providing leadership and a framework of support for local PPIFs, and representing patient and public perspectives in national policy.
- A statutory duty on NHS organizations to consult and involve patients and the public in the planning of services, proposals for changes in services and decisions about how services operate.
- The creation of Foundation Trusts from 2003 onwards, which established a further form of public involvement and accountability, with individual members of the public (and staff) able to join these organizations as members and elect representatives on to their governing bodies.

These arrangements were strongly oriented towards healthcare services rather than public health. PALS and ICAS were focused almost wholly on personal healthcare services (although some of these services had an important prevention or health promotion dimension). PPIFs, especially those based in provider Trusts, were overwhelmingly concerned with healthcare services. Those based in PCTs had a wider remit to promote and support public involvement in wider issues of health locally and to represent public views on matters affecting health. Even here, however, the principal focus remained on health services. The national body, the CPPIH, tried to incorporate a broader public health perspective, in line with its statutory functions (which included the promotion of the public's involvement in decisions affecting their health). But it was hampered by resource constraints and political pressures from the Department of Health to concentrate its efforts on healthcare.

Despite these reforms, patient and public involvement remained a low priority for the NHS (Health Committee, 2003, 2007). It was an underresourced, highly fragmented system confusing to the public and staff, and dominated by professional and management concerns (Baggott, 2005; Hogg, 2009). There was also disquiet about the independence of the new bodies. Meanwhile, Foundation Trusts were viewed as having a mixed effect on the accountability of hospitals to the public, while appearing to enhance the legitimacy of these of these bodies relative to other NHS organizations (Allen et al., 2012). The CPPIH was heavily criticized for lacking leadership and failing to provide effective support for the PPIFs. The legitimacy and credibility of the PPIFs was challenged, amid criticism of their cost, low public profile, overbureaucratic nature, lack of representativeness, limited engagement with the public and patients, and lack of influence over the NHS (Health Committee, 2007; Healthcare Commission, 2009; Hogg, 2009). Some were more optimistic about the longer term potential of PPIFs (Martin, 2008), and even critics felt that with time they might have evolved into more effective organizations (Health Committee, 2007; Warwick, 2007). Despite reservations about the impact of further restructuring, the government abolished the CPPIH and PPIFs in 2008, replacing the latter with Local Involvement Networks (LINks).

LINks

LINks were funded and established by local authorities with social services responsibilities (that is, county councils and unitary authorities). Local authorities received a non-ring-fenced grant from central government for this purpose. Their remit included social care as well as health services. They were smaller in number (150 were created, compared with approximately 400 PPIFs) and focused on a geographical area rather than an NHS organization. Their key functions were: to promote and support the involvement of people in the commissioning, provision and scrutiny of health and social care; to enable people to monitor and review the commissioning and provision of local health and social care services; to obtain the views of people about their health and social care needs and experiences; to present these views to those responsible for commissioning, providing, managing and scrutinizing health and social care services; and to make recommendations about service improvements.

LINks had a number of duties and powers. Like CHCs and PPIFs, they were required to produce an annual report on their activities. Like PPIFs, they were able to refer matters to HOSCs and were granted rights of entry and view to healthcare premises where services were provided (incidentally, CHCs had similar rights, but these were more restricted). LINks were also permitted to enter and inspect social care premises (with some exceptions, such as children's homes) and independent providers of state-funded care. Similar to PPIFs, and CHCs before them, LINks were able to make requests for information from, and to report or make recommendations to, local service providers. Unlike PPIFs and CHCs, membership of LINks was not prescribed by central government. This enabled them to develop more flexibly, to involve a wider range of individuals and groups. An advantage of LINks over PPIFs was that they (like CHCs) covered areas, rather than institutions. This meant that they could represent local people on a range of issues that cut across the responsibilities of specific service commissioners and providers. The extension of their remit to social care meant that they had greater scope for covering the interface between healthcare, social care and public health. This created a possibility that LINks might become more involved in matters of health and well-being, service integration and coordination. Moreover, given that LINks were area-based, it was thought that they would develop a closer relationship with HOSCs and together take a greater interest in factors affecting people's health.

One of the main disadvantages was that LINks were local authority-funded, creating potential conflicts of interest (as councils were also responsible for commissioning and providing social care services). Councils were not permitted to run LINks directly, but had to commission them from a 'host' organization, responsible for organizing and developing their key functions (such as providing administrative support, communications, reporting and recruitment of members). A number of voluntary organizations, including social enterprises, acted as hosts (and had previously undertaken a similar function for PPIFs). Although there were regulations on the establishment, duties and powers of LINks, there was no blueprint for how they should operate. In 2006, the NHS National Centre for Involvement was established by the Department of Health (in partnership with Warwick University) to provide guidance for LINks and to promote and support patient and public involvement within the NHS, but this was closed down in 2009.

Notwithstanding arguments for local flexibility and autonomy, there was concern about a variation in the quality of LINks and their impact. The Centre for Public Scrutiny (2011) found that although the majority of LINks reported making 'more progress', there was considerable variation in their impact, their engagement with communities and their relationship with other bodies. There were also differences in achievement across different areas of activity (relationships with social care providers being a particular concern). An official analysis of LINks annual reports for 2010–11 (DH, 2011c) estimated that 31 per cent of the total number of reports submitted by LINks to relevant health and social care services, and 50 per cent of their referrals to HOSCs, led to service changes. A further analysis, covering the period 2011–12, found that these figures had fallen to 21 per cent and 30 per cent, respectively (DH, 2013b). In both reports, around a quarter of LINks that reported on their outcomes claimed that five or more service changes had resulted from their reports or recommendations. Even so, how significant these changes were is unknown, and it is it impossible to verify the impact that LINks had on actual decisions (DH, 2013b).

A second issue was the limited engagement between LINks and the public. Awareness of LINks was low – in one survey, over half of patients were unaware of their existence (Patients Association, 2011). The Department of Health (DH, 2011c) estimated that, in 2010–11, approximately 153,000 people participated in LINks in some way. The number of active participants, however, was much less, at over 10,000 (although this compared favourably with the official estimate of 3,977 PPIF members; CPPIH, 2008). In the following year, the total number of participants fell by 17 per cent, although that of active participants increased by 7 per cent (DH, 2013b). Although there were no data to confirm that LINks were any more or less representative of their communities than PPIFs, it was widely acknowledged that they similarly struggled to achieve a balanced membership with regard to age, social class and other social characteristics.

Another problem with the new system was weak accountability between local authorities, LINks and the host organizations. Moreover, the whole system of public and user involvement in health lacked coherence and stature, and this weakened the accountability of the NHS to local people (LGA, 2008). Indeed, the Mid Staffordshire Foundation Trust Public Inquiry (2013) was highly critical of the weaknesses of PPIFs and LINks (and local government health scrutiny bodies), labelling them 'a conspicuous failure' (p. 74).

There is no solid evidence on whether LINks focused more on public health matters than their predecessor bodies had. There is anecdotal evidence that some LINks examined public health issues, particularly those related to health promotion services. A trawl through individual LINk websites and annual reports reveals activities across a range of issues including mental health, health inequalities, sexual health services and healthy eating. Efforts by some LINks to engage with 'hard to reach' groups may have had important public health implications by highlighting neglected health needs. However, the picture is broadly similar to what happened previously with CHCs and PPIFs: some took an interest in prevention and public health, but the majority were overwhelmingly focused on care and treatment services.

Other developments under New Labour

Finally in this section, it is important to note other relevant developments during the last years of New Labour. First, 'World Class Commissioning' (see Chapter 3) set out a number of areas where commissioning organizations (that is, PCTs) had to develop skills and capacity (such as leadership, strategy development and contracting). Importantly, these included 'engagement' (including engagement with the public and service users). Moreover, the vision of World Class Commissioning was not confined to healthcare services but included health improvement and reducing health inequalities. One of the key 'competences' PCTs were expected to achieve was to 'proactively seek and build continuous and meaningful engagement with the public and patients, to shape services and improve health' (DH, 2007b, p. 16). There are some indications that World Class Commissioning did help to improve the status of patient and public involvement within PCTs, but little evidence that local communities were able to influence decisions (Picker Institute, 2009).

Second, engagement with the public and users was relevant to the government's health and well-being commissioning strategic framework (DH, 2007c). This required local government and the NHS (via PCTs) to engage in Joint Strategic Needs Assessments (JSNAs; see Chapters 3 and 4) and emphasized community engagement.

Third, the Darzi Review of the NHS highlighted the importance of preventing illness and empowering patients to participate in healthcare decisions (Cm 7432, 2008). The focus was mainly on the individuals' role in self-care, adopting healthier lifestyles and making choices about their own care. However, Darzi acknowledged that the voluntary sector had a role in service planning and provision, and that public views should be taken into account when formulating strategic plans. Importantly, Darzi recommended that NHS bodies should be given a duty to have regard to an NHS constitution setting out principles, rights and pledges. The constitution, introduced in 2009 and subsequently revised (DH, 2010c, 2012d) included rights to consultation and involvement in service planning and delivery (discussed in more detail below) along with two pledges: to provide people with the information needed to influence and scrutinize the planning and delivery of services; and a commitment to working in partnership with patients, relatives, carers and their representatives.

Fourth, the statutory right to consultation and involvement (set out in Section 11 of the Health and Social Care Act 2001 and consolidated in Section 242 of the National Health Service Act 2006) was amended. The original legislation required NHS organizations (PCTs, Strategic Health Authorities [SHAs], NHS Trusts and Foundation Trusts) to involve and consult current and potential service users in the planning of services provision, the development and consideration of proposals for changes in the way services were provided, and decisions made by NHS organizations affecting the operation of services. The duty was regarded as too wide-ranging and unspecific, and easy to evade in practice (Health Committee, 2007). It was subjected to judicial review and subsequently revised by the Local Government and Public Involvement in Health Act 2007. The new legislation stated that relevant NHS bodies:

> must make arrangements, as respects health services for which it is responsible, which secure that users of those services, whether directly or through representatives, are involved (whether by being consulted, or provided with information, or in other ways) in (a) the planning of the provision of those services, (b) the development and consideration of proposals for changes in the way those services are provided, and (c) decisions to be made by that body affecting the operation of those services.

Users were defined as actual and potential users. However, there was a restriction on the scope for involvement for proposals in relation to (b) and (c), where the duty to involve only applied if the proposal or decision related to the manner in which services were delivered (that is, concerned the point of delivery and not the means of delivery) or the range of services delivered. This was criticized for blocking user involvement in decisions to transfer services to non-NHS bodies. Critics also argued that public and user involvement should be mandatory in other areas, such as health needs assessment and setting health priorities. The legislation did, however, create an additional requirement on SHAs and PCTs to prepare reports on consultation processes with regard to commissioning and other relevant decisions, and on the influence of such consultations on decisions.

The Cameron government and patient and public involvement

The system was altered further in the light of the Coalition's NHS reforms (Cm 7881, 2010; see Chapter 4). The new government proposed replacing LINks with local healthwatch organizations and creating a new national body, Healthwatch England. In addition, duties were placed on other health bodies to involve patients and the public in their work. These plans were eventually enacted by the Health and Social Care Act 2012. During the passage of this legislation, a number of amendments were made to strengthen the provisions on patient and public involvement, arising from recommendations by the NHS Future Forum (2011a, 2011b; see Chapter 4) and pressure from patients' associations, other voluntary organizations and some health service and local government organizations.

Healthwatch England was established as a statutory committee of the Care Quality Commission (CQC), the body responsible for inspecting, investigating and monitoring standards of health and social care in England. It was given powers to recommend that CQC carry out specific investigations of services where problems had been identified. To strengthen the links between the CQC and Healthwatch England, it was decided to appoint the chair of the latter to the CQC board. There was, however, concern about the location of Healthwatch England within the CQC, and safeguards were introduced to protect its independence and strengthen accountability. It was made clear that Healthwatch England could not contain a majority of members drawn from the CQC. Provision was also made for guidance to be issued by the Secretary of State on managing potential conflicts of interest between Healthwatch England and the CQC. A requirement was placed on the CQC to respond formally in writing to requests from Healthwatch England. In an effort to maintain the profile of Healthwatch England and strengthen accountability, it was added to the list of health bodies that the Secretary of State had to keep under review. In the interests of transparency, Healthwatch England meetings were made open to the public.

Healthwatch England functions include advising several bodies about the views of service users and the public, regarding their need for and experiences of health and social care services, the standards of these services and how these might be improved. These bodies include the CQC, the Secretary of State for Health, Monitor (the regulator of markets and competition in the newly reformed NHS), local authorities and NHS England. Duties have been placed on some of these bodies to consult with Healthwatch England on specific matters (for example, NHS England must consult Healthwatch England when formulating its guidance to Clinical Commissioning Groups [CCGs], while the Secretary of State for Health must consult it before setting out the mandate for the NHS). Another key function of Healthwatch England is to provide advice and assistance to local healthwatch organizations (discussed further below). Furthermore, Healthwatch England is empowered to issue general guidance to local authorities on their healthwatch arrangements and can write to individual local authorities if it has concerns about their healthwatch service. To strengthen the links between the national and local bodies, the government agreed that up to four members of Healthwatch England's governing body (a third of its membership) should be drawn from local healthwatch bodies.

Local healthwatch organizations, like LINks before them, are funded by county councils and unitary local authorities through a non-ring-fenced grant from central government. However, local healthwatch organizations differ from LINks in that they are corporate bodies and may employ their own staff. The government initially intended that local healthwatch would be statutory bodies. However, it later decided that while local healthwatch organizations would indeed have statutory powers, they would be established as social enterprises (see Box 7.1). In addition, local healthwatch organizations were permitted to subcontract some of their functions to other bodies (which did not have to be social enterprises). Although social enterprises were already involved in supporting LINks and previously PPIFs (as host organizations), this U-turn took most observers by surprise. The government emphasized that local areas needed more flexibility in establishing their local healthwatch, and that the creation of statutory bodies would entail a more prescriptive and centralized approach. It also wanted to encourage social enterprise as part of its Big Society agenda. Critics argued that local healthwatch organizations would not be taken as seriously by service providers if they were not statutory bodies. They also feared that social enterprises might not be able to represent the public and might not necessarily act in the public interest, and that the subcontracting of local healthwatch functions would undermine the coherence of the new system.

Some safeguards were introduced by the government in the form of statutory regulations. The meaning of a social enterprise was clarified (to ensure that at least 50 per cent of profits of the organization had to be reinvested to secure benefits for the community). The regulations also enabled particular voluntary organizations, such as registered charities, to be classified as a social enterprise for the purpose of establishing local healthwatch organizations (thus allowing charities to provide local healthwatch services). In addition, the government prescribed various requirements regarding procedures, decision-making and other matters that must be reflected in local healthwatch arrangements. For example, it specified that local healthwatch bodies must include lay people and volunteers in their governance arrangements. To clarify local healthwatch responsibilities with regard to representation of the whole community, the Health and Social Care Act 2012 Section 182(8) had earlier defined local people as 'people who live in the local authority's area; people to whom care services are being or may be provided in that area; and people from that area to whom care services are being provided in any place, and who are (taken together) representative of the people' (in these categories).

More controversially, the ability of healthwatch to engage in political activity was restricted (to activities incidental to its main objective of benefiting the community). This was seen by some as an effort to 'gag' local healthwatch bodies and prevent them from lobbying to influence public policy (Calkin, 2013). The government later clarified that the intention was not to stop local healthwatch bodies from raising concerns or advocating changes in policy or the law, providing this was based on evidence. It was to prevent these bodies from aligning themselves to a particular party, making political activities their main activity and having policy changes as their primary purpose.

Compared with LINks, local healthwatch organizations acquired additional powers and responsibilities. These included providing information and advice to individuals about access to health and social care services and choice regarding these services. They were also charged with providing (or signposting) independent advocacy support for complaints about health and social care services. Local healthwatch bodies are also empowered to refer matters to Healthwatch England and the CQC for further investigation. Requirements on bodies to respond to healthwatch reports and recommendations within a certain period were extended to providers of children's social services. However, the original 20-day response time can now be extended for matters deemed complex (for example, where a local healthwatch report or recommendation relates to several different bodies). There was disappointment that specific duties in the Health and Social Care Act 2012 to compel all health and social care bodies to provide information to local healthwatch bodies were not brought into force. Healthwatch bodies must instead use Freedom of Information requests, which may be refused and can involve significant costs. The government did, however, bring in regulations to compel private providers to respond to requests for information from local healthwatch bodies (subject to certain restrictions, such as confidentiality).

In addition, local healthwatch bodies were given a new role in relation to public health, inequalities and integrated care. Local healthwatch organizations are represented on the new Health and Wellbeing Boards for their area and must be involved in the JSNA and the development of the Joint Health and Wellbeing Strategy (JHWS) (see Chapters 3 and 4).

The Health and Social Care Act 2012 also placed duties on other bodies. NHS England has a statutory duty to promote the involvement of individual patients and carers in decisions about the provision of health services to them, and a broader requirement to ensure public and patient involvement in health service planning and commissioning activities. CCGs must promote patient and public involvement in service provision, planning and commissioning, and include information about how they will discharge these duties in their commissioning plans and report on their activities in their annual reports. Interestingly, the initial legislation confined such duties of involvement to situations where there was a 'significant' impact on services. Under pressure, the government removed the word 'significant'. It also strengthened the duties of NHS England and the CCGs with regard to the NHS Constitution (which contains rights and pledges on involvement) and in patient and carer involvement in decisions about themselves.

Following other amendments, CCGs must now set out a statement of principles and the arrangements for patient and public involvement in their published constitutions. These must be assessed by NHS England for compliance with patient and public involvement standards before they become operational. In addition, NHS England must assess as part of its annual assessment of CCGs how well they are undertaking patient and public involvement. NHS England must also include a section on patient and public involvement in its annual plan and report (which the Secretary of State is required to report upon and lay before Parliament). CCGs must heed guidance from NHS England on individual patient involvement in service provision, as well as public involvement in planning and commissioning. To strengthen public accountability, CCGs are required to meet in public (except on commercially sensitive issues) and must have at least two lay members on their board. In addition, duties and requirements on patient and public involvement have been imposed on Monitor. Furthermore, commissioners, providers, managers and scrutiny bodies must give proper regard to local healthwatch reports and recommendations.

At the time of writing, the new system of patient and public involvement is being implemented. Healthwatch England was established in 2012, and local healthwatch organizations officially began their work in April 2013 (although there were delays in establishing local healthwatch bodies in some areas). However, a number of 'pathfinder' bodies were established prior to this, to provide a foundation for the new system and enable lessons for future practice. The experience of pathfinders (LGA and Centre for Public Scrutiny, 2012; LGA et al., 2012a, 2012b), coupled with further details about how the new system is intended to operate, also led to further criticism.

First, there was disquiet about resource allocation. There was concern that the refusal to ring-fence their funding could leave them short of funds (notably a number of LINks did not receive their full allocation under the previous system, which also was not ring-fenced; see DH, 2011c, 2013b). The overall amount that the government was intending to provide for local healthwatch organizations was also criticized as being insufficient, especially in the light of additional responsibilities they had acquired. The government initially agreed to provide £27 million of baseline funding per annum plus additional resources for setting up local healthwatch bodies and for their additional roles (amounting to £11.5 million for each of the first two years of their operation). Subsequently, following complaints, the additional element was increased to £16.5 million per annum. Despite this more generous settlement, the average amount allocated to each local healthwatch body remained small (approximately £280,000) relative to the tasks they were expected to perform.

Second, there were fears about the impact of reorganization (of both the system of patient and public involvement and the NHS in general). Some were concerned that the new reforms failed to build on the legacy of the previous public involvement system. For example, there was a risk that existing volunteers and lay people involved in LINks could become marginalized and disaffected, and as a result might not participate in healthwatch organizations (LGA et al., 2012b). In some areas, there was a lack of engagement with voluntary organizations in the design and development of local healthwatch, despite their experience of previous systems of patient and public involvement and their expertise in volunteer management, organizational governance and accessing 'hard to reach' groups (LGA et al., 2012b). By creating entirely new bodies, existing momentum could be lost, and this meant that capacity would have to be rebuilt.

Third, there were strong views that the new system of patient and public involvement had not been fully based on an understanding of the failures of previous systems. Indeed, previous research into LINks had identified shortcomings in capacity and had recommended a coordinated programme of information and support for the new organizations (Centre for Public Scrutiny, 2011), a view echoed by others (LGA et al., 2012b). It was also believed that the new system (like the previous ones) lacked a public profile and would need time and resources to establish one (Patients Association, 2011; LGA et al., 2012b). Moreover, it was feared that, notwithstanding the duties and responsibilities imposed on NHS England, CCGs and Monitor, the complexity of implementing the wider NHS reforms would distract them from the task of building genuine patient and public involvement, and that in practice this would have low priority.

Concerns persisted about the coherence of local healthwatch, resulting from the decision to create a role for social enterprises and allow subcontracting of its functions. Furthermore, it was acknowledged that much more needed to be done to build effective links between the scrutiny functions of local authorities, Health and Wellbeing Boards and local healthwatch organizations. This would not occur by chance but required good working practices and the development of strong mutual relationships based on trust (LGA and Centre for Public Scrutiny, 2012). There was also a range of outstanding concerns about the independence of the new bodies (including Healthwatch England) and about their powers (particularly with regard to influencing policy and securing information, already referred to). Finally, it was widely believed that the primary focus of patient and public involvement remained upon health services, although the inclusion of duties to involve local healthwatch and the public in the preparation of JSNAs and JHWSs was seen as providing opportunities to strengthen involvement in public health issues.

Other aspects of community participation in health and well-being

Community participation in local government and other relevant programmes

The Coalition's plans to transfer key public health functions from the NHS to local government offered an opportunity to strengthen community involvement. Local authorities had already increased their efforts to involve the public, undertaking surveys and focus groups, establishing advisory forums and citizens' juries, and engaging in consultation with their communities (Lowndes and Pratchett, 2001a, 2001b). In addition, community participation was mandatory in some regeneration and welfare programmes (such as Sure Start and the Neighbourhood Renewal Strategy) where local authorities had an important role. Local authorities also engaged in community involvement through their leadership of Local Strategic Partnerships (LSPs; see Chapter 3). As well as seeking to coordinate policies, strategies and services across local agencies, LSPs had the potential to improve community involvement across local agencies by promoting good practice and avoiding unnecessary duplication. However, they were unable to improve the coherence of community involvement as much as envisaged due to their limited powers and resources (Taylor, 2006; Barnes et al., 2007; DCLG, 2011a), Indeed, they often added to the problem of duplication and consultation 'fatigue' (see below).

Community participation in local government attracted similar criticisms to that in the NHS. There was much variability, with some councils being much more committed and effective than others. Shortcomings included: lack of agreement on the purpose of participation, limited capacity for public engagement, poor feedback to communities, tokenism and a lack of empowerment, and 'consultation fatigue', where the same council – and in some cases other local agencies – undertook similar consultations in a short period of time within the same community or group of users (Select Committee on Public Administration, 2001; Cook, 2002; Needham, 2002; Skidmore et al., 2006; Taylor, 2006; DCLG,

2008). Research demonstrated that public and user involvement tended to reflect management agendas and generated much scepticism about the process (Barnes et al., 2007). There was also particular difficulty in engaging with some social groups and users, such as children and young people, other vulnerable persons, deprived communities and some ethnic groups (Gilchrist, 2006; Taylor, 2006). Indeed, the legitimacy of community involvement was often disputed, given the dependence on the 'usual suspects', a relatively small number of highly committed individuals with the time and resources to get involved (Cook, 2002; Gilchrist, 2006). On a more positive note, community involvement was sometimes able to contribute to policy and service delivery and may have had a positive effect on social cohesion (Barnes et al., 2007; Burton et al., 2008). Much, however, appeared to rest on the design of engagement processes, the attitudes and expectations of public authorities and the community, an acknowledgement of the diversity of communities, and levels of support and resources for engagement processes.

So far the discussion has centred on community participation in England. The other countries of the UK have also introduced processes for involving the public and users in policy, planning and service provision. These are discussed further in Box 5.3.

Box 5.3	Public and user participation in Scotland, Wales and Northern Ireland

In Scotland, Community Planning Partnerships (see Chapter 3) bring together local public sector and voluntary organizations, and produce community plans and joint health improvement plans for their area. Public authorities and partnerships actively involve the public and service users and also engage in community development (where the Scottish Community Development Centre sets standards). There is also a separate system of public and patient involvement. Each health board (which has a duty to ensure patient and public involvement) has at least one Community Health Partnership, which has a remit for integrating services, improving partnership working, improving health and reducing health inequalities (although these are in the process of being replaced; see Chapter 3). Currently, each Community Health Partnership has a public partnership forum through which local people and voluntary organizations can be engaged in planning, decision-making and service development. These forums replaced the previous system of local health councils (similar to CHCs in England and Wales) in 2005. A national body, the Scottish Health Council, was established to monitor, support and review patient and public involvement in health matters. This body is a subcommittee of Healthcare Improvement Scotland (similar to the CQC in England). The Scottish Health Council has local offices located in each health board area, which support public partnership forums and NHS bodies on patient and public involvement issues and monitor processes locally. In 2010, this body was reorganized, following criticism of its structure, to enable it to focus more strongly on its core functions (see Scottish Health Council, 2013). It should be noted that Scottish health boards also contain lay representatives, and the Scottish government has recently experimented with direct election of members to these boards. However, an interim report found low turn-outs, apathy and higher costs than predicted (Greer et al., 2011).

In Wales, too, efforts have been made to improve public and user engagement and community development. In 2001, Communities First, a programme funded by the Welsh Assembly government, was launched to fund community development workers in the most disadvantaged communities. These teams support initiatives that involve health promotion and have an ethos of partnership working with other agencies. A national community development body (Community Development Cymru) was established in 2002. Following on from this, a new national strategic framework for community development was introduced in 2007. In addition, there are grant schemes for developing capacity and capability in public health improvement in the voluntary and community sector. There is some evidence that these schemes have led to greater opportunities for community engagement, but little evidence of an impact on statutory agencies (see Adamson and Bromily, 2008). Specifically with regard to patient and public involvement, Wales retained CHCs and strengthened their role. They are currently facing a new round of reforms (Welsh Government, 2012). The Welsh Government has also produced good practice guidance for NHS bodies in Wales (National Assembly for Wales and Office of Public Management, 2002; Welsh Assembly Government, 2003b). Local health boards and NHS Trusts in Wales are required to consult and involve the public and patients, and must self-assess their activities in this field (and are also assessed through the NHS Wales performance framework). There is no evidence to suggest that the model for patient and public involvement in Wales is any more or less effective than that adopted in England (Hughes et al., 2009).

In Northern Ireland, community development has been a key priority, partly because of its importance in building a cohesive and equal community in the light of the 'troubles'. There is a Community Development and Health Network, which supports and informs those working in this field and promotes community development. Northern Ireland also has a system of patient and public involvement that was reformed a few years ago. In 2009, a Patient and Client Council was created, replacing the four Health and Social Care Councils in Northern Ireland. The functions of the new body are: to provide information and advice on health and social services issues, to help complainants, to monitor the quality of local services, to work with local groups and help them to articulate their views, to act on behalf of the public to improve services, to survey public views on services, and to represent the public's interest in consultations on health and social services, and regularly visit health and social service facilities.

Community development

It is one thing to build a partnership with the community by listening to views, concerns and ideas regarding policy and service development. However, this is unlikely to lead to the empowerment of the public or service users and does not engage people improving their own health (Skidmore et al., 2006; NICE, 2008c). In order to achieve this, public authorities (and their partners in the voluntary sector; see Chapter 6) must engage in community development – defined in relation to health as 'active engagement with a defined group of people over an extended period of time in order to identify and tackle some of the social, economic, environmental and political issues that determine their health and quality of life' (Naidoo and Wills, 2005, p. 123).

Community development involves professionals, lay people, organizations and informal groups working in partnership to improve health and well-being. It has been described as a form of health promotion (Gilchrist, 2003), rooted in an approach that places great emphasis on empowerment, partnership, informal networks and respect for lay perspectives. It seeks to build the capacity of the community and is based on a holistic model of health (Amos, 2002). A further development of this approach is to emphasize the 'assets' of the community (rather than its 'deficits' and 'needs'), to develop and utilize the existing capacity and resources of the community to improve health and well-being (IDeA, 2010). An emphasis on community development does not mean that professionals or public bodies are absent or relegated to a minor role in promoting health and well-being. On the contrary, their activities are crucial in supporting the community to fulfil its potential. In addition, voluntary and community organizations, sometimes funded by public authorities, play a key role in establishing the networks that support community development work.

Community development is found in many areas of public health and well-being, including smoking cessation, healthy eating, the promotion of physical exercise and addressing social determinants of health (Ritchie et al., 2004; Handsley, 2007; Morgan and Popay, 2007). Government programmes such as Sure Start, Health Action Zones, Healthy Living Centres, regeneration and sustainable development programmes, as well as specific community health projects funded by government (for example, those within the Communities for Health and Healthy Towns programmes) have acknowledged its value. However, government and public authorities have often been criticized for not pursuing a genuine community development approach (Naidoo and Wills, 2005; Mackereth, 2006; Bowles, 2010), relying too much on a 'top-down' initiatives and professionally dominant approaches. Other criticisms (of both community development in general, and its application to health) are that projects are too piecemeal, ad hoc and short term, too small scale and fragmented, and not properly evaluated (see Bowles, 2010). Valuable lessons about what is effective, and what is not, have not been learned. Such projects have also been criticized for focusing too much on changing personal behaviour and not enough on overcoming obstacles to effective policy and practice (Amos, 2002). More fundamentally, government-backed programmes are criticized for failing to challenge structures of inequality and disadvantage that underpin health problems facing many communities (Crawshaw et al., 2003). A lack of strategic focus has been identified. This has led to inadequate and short-term funding. Paradoxically, given the stated importance of community development to reform agendas such as choice, personalization and community participation, much community development work is precarious and seemingly undervalued by statutory authorities (Bowles, 2010).

Community development can produce social change. But government (both central and local) is concerned that this might be difficult to contain or manage. It might also lead to excessive or unrealistic expectations. Government prefers top-down initiatives that can demonstrate some impact on individuals but that do not build into social movements for radical change. In 2009, the Labour government allocated £75 million to Change4Life (C4L), a three-year programme, aimed at getting people to adopt a healthier lifestyle. Given the high profile of the campaign, it achieved high recognition from the public and the initial key target group (mothers with children under 11 years of age): 87 per cent of the target group were aware of the campaign, and 413,000 families signed up to the programme. Over 44,000 families continued to interact with programme six months after joining. Follow-up surveys reported that three out of 10 mothers made changes to their children's lifestyles as a direct result of the campaign (DH, 2010d). Although this sounds impressive, there is no hard evidence that the programme either empowered individuals or led to sustained changes in lifestyles. Moreover, the programme focused on changing the behaviour of individuals and families. It did not challenge the socioeconomic structures and other barriers that inhibit healthy eating and exercise within communities (such as junk food advertising, the high prices of healthy foods for poor families and the closure of sports facilities and green spaces).

However, it is possible that C4L might have a longer term impact. First, a number of projects involved more focused efforts to address the environment in which people made choices, for example working with local retailers to improve access to, promotion of and consumption of fruit and vegetables (see Chapter 7). Work with sports organizations to encourage participation and increase physical activity also looked promising. Second, the C4L 'brand' was used by local health promotion agencies across the NHS, local government and voluntary sectors. Many existing and new activities were rebadged, providing a focal point for promoting local health and well-being interventions and acting as a catalyst for drawing together local policies and resources (for example, see www.sheffieldc4l. org.uk). Some areas appointed C4L coordinators to strengthen partnership working and community engagement. Third, C4L created a network of community champions, people who agreed to sign up and become more closely involved in health promotion activities. While this new network was initially underutilized, it had potential for further development, which the Coalition government was keen to develop in the context of its 'Big Society' idea. Fourth, other nationally funded demonstration and pilot projects were linked to the C4L brand (Box 5.4).

Box 5.4   **Examples of community health programmes and projects**

Community health projects have arisen from a variety of sources. Some emerged out of regeneration programmes, others out of Healthy City initiatives, Health Action Zones, Healthy Living Centres, Sure Start and others (see Chapter 3). In some cases, initiatives developed out of local agendas, such as anti-poverty strategies, housing improvement plans or wider community development initiatives. This has led to a fragmented, piecemeal and ad hoc approach. Funding for projects has tended to be short term, with little evaluation or learning from past projects, and an absence of a strategic framework. The Department of Health sought to address this by funding the Communities for Health programme in 2004. Starting with a number of pilot projects, the programme lasted seven years, channelling additional funding to local authorities working in partnership with the NHS and the voluntary and private sectors. The programme aimed to engage communities in their own health and develop their capacity for supporting individual behavioural change to healthier lifestyles, build partnerships between organizations and communities, and develop innovative practices for community-based health improvements. The projects funded were diverse, reflecting a desire to allow local authorities and their partners to develop projects with their communities in a flexible way. There was an emphasis on improving health, reducing health inequalities, strengthening partnership working across sectors and communities, building capacity, basing interventions on evidence, evaluating interventions, sharing information and learning lessons, promoting innovation and ensuring sustainable practice.

Three hundred and sixty activities and interventions were funded by the programme, across over 80 local authority areas. The projects focused on a range of issues including health inequalities, smoking, obesity, alcohol problems, sexual health and mental health. Some focused on whole populations, others on specific groups such as children, women, men, ethnic minorities or older people. Some projects supported the development of overarching health and well-being strategies by local authorities (for example, Nottingham's Decade of Better Health and Liverpool's Health and Wellbeing framework). Others aimed to develop strategic approaches to particular issues, such as physical exercise (Blackburn and Darwen's Re:fresh initiative) or breastfeeding (Coventry). In addition, many projects adopted practical ways to attain further strategic objectives, such as community development. Some areas (notably Nottingham, Sandwell and Croydon) provided training for their employees or for members of the public to take on health promotion roles (for example, to motivate others by acting as 'health champions', or as 'buddies' for people needing support to access services or change their lifestyles).

An evaluation of the programme was positive, finding that it raised understanding of the determinants of health among local public service managers and produced stronger partnership working between local agencies (LGA, 2011a, 2011b). It also promoted a more positive approach to health improvement and well-being, rather than a narrower perspective on preventing disease. In so doing, it was able to engage those outside the health sector more successfully than might have otherwise been the case. The provision of resources through local authorities was viewed as beneficial because it gave them an important leadership role and a sense of ownership. It also enabled alignment of the programme with other initiatives in related areas such as housing, regeneration, training and skills development, and the environment. The flexibility of the funding regime was seen as encouraging diversity, flexibility and innovation. Importance was placed on the role of local coordinators and regional networks in giving the programme coherence and ensuring that learning experiences were shared.

The programme generated important lessons for community-based initiatives. These were: that wider determinants of health can be tackled through collaboration between local services; that opportunities for user involvement and co-production must be maximized; that user perspectives must be at the centre of design for health improvement; that objectives should be set to improve population health and reduce health inequalities; that mainstream services need to build knowledge of public health among the workforce (not just in the NHS but in local government and the voluntary sector); that messages about health improvement need to be kept simple and emphasize their rationale; and finally that those commissioning public health services need to ensure that potential providers (especially in the voluntary and community sectors) have the capacity and opportunity to tender for work.

The Communities for Health programme appears to have achieved some success, most notably in strengthening interagency relationships and stimulating community development networks in health. But the programme could have been subject to more robust evaluation. There is little evidence of improved health outcomes (although some projects have been able to demonstrate improvements such as increased rates of usage of facilities and services). A further problem was that the funding for the programme was short term and there was considerable uncertainty over how long the funding would last, which inhibited planning. Funding for the programme ended in 2011, although some projects have continued with funding from local agencies. Other initiatives have also been pursued, with the aim of involving communities more closely in health improvement. For example, Altogether Better, a programme initially consisting of projects in the Yorkshire and Humber Region and funded by the Big Lottery Fund, focused on strengthening civic participation in health through volunteers. It has recruited and trained 17,000 health champions (including workplace champions) to promote healthy lifestyles in their communities. These champions engaged in a range of activities including informal interactions with other people as part of their daily lives, providing more intensive support for some individuals, and organizing or leading activities and events (such as walks and other healthy activities, presentations on health matters, and running voluntary and community groups). An evaluation of the programme found that champions reported a number of benefits both for themselves (increased confidence and self-esteem, a healthier lifestyle, improved mental health and well-being, and better knowledge and awareness of health issues) and for the wider community (White et al., 2010).

Conclusion

In recent years, there has been a strong and growing rationale for community and service user involvement in public health and well-being. Recent governments have acknowledged this, and it has been reflected in both policy and specific programmes. However, efforts to strengthen participation in this area (and in the NHS and public services more generally) have been confused by a lack of clarity of aims and inconsistent terminology. What is clear though is an overwhelming desire on the part of government and NHS organizations to control and manage community participation. This has been characterized by a top-down approach, a focus on limited and often cursory consultation and (with the exception of a few well-documented examples) a lack of community empowerment. In addition, there has been an attempt to restrict the sphere of community participation and public accountability. This negative approach, coupled with a failure to join up initiatives with a broader community development approach, led to a reactive and piecemeal system. This situation was not helped by continuing weaknesses in patient and public involvment systems (related to funding, powers and independence) and successive reforms that caused disruption while not building sufficiently on previous experience. Problems in this field have been further compounded by poor-quality evaluation and a failure to learn from good practice.

A further problem has been the primary focus of community participation on health services (and in particular diagnosis, care and treatment). One can argue that most community participation on public health and well-being has taken place on programmes outside or at least on the margins of what might be regarded as conventional health policy (for example, regeneration schemes, child welfare programmes and community-based health programmes). It remains to be seen whether the latest incarnation of public participation in health, Healthwatch, fares any better than its predecessors in promoting community participation, securing public accountability and influencing matters of public health and well-being.

Another point is that much of the focus of community participation in health has been upon public and patient representation within institutional structures. Although it is indeed important that efforts are made to ensure that health policy-makers and service providers are responsive and accountable through systems of patient and user representation, and that lay expertise and experiential knowledge are incorporated into decision-making, other less formal forms of participation should be encouraged. People can also be influential as 'everyday makers', getting involved in health promotion and disease prevention through personal, voluntary activities (such as acting as health champions).

Despite the rhetoric surrounding community participation, policies and programmes have in reality been strongly influenced by a need to demonstrate that there is a new form of governance that welcomes public involvement, while in practice holding tightly on to the reins of power. As the Marmot Report argued, community engagement practices must go beyond routine consultations. They require changes to power structures and must remove barriers to participation. This requires a different kind of leadership and management than has hitherto been practised (Strategic Review of Health Inequalities in England, 2010). One of the key shortcomings has been the failure to build adequate capacity needed to expand community participation. As will be shown in the next chapter, the voluntary sector has received support and resources, and this has been used for community development work, but even here there have been problems.

Failures in community participation are damaging, as they breed cynicism and place burdens on people without benefit. Tokenism may succeed in the short term, and enable policy-makers and local agencies to create an illusion of representation and accountability. But this is only a temporary solution and causes long-term damage. It creates disappointment and discontent, undermines partnerships with users and the wider community, stifles co-production and ultimately corrodes the legitimacy on which public services depend.

6 Partnerships with the voluntary sector

Introduction

The voluntary sector has been identified as vital in securing greater community involvement in health and well-being, and improving public services in this field. This chapter explores key policy developments affecting the voluntary sector and the implications for partnership working in health and well-being. It begins with a discussion of the nature of the voluntary sector in general, including a brief historical context, key concepts and definitions, and indicators of its size and scope. This is followed by an analysis of the policies adopted by previous and current governments towards the sector. The next section considers in more detail the role of voluntary organizations in health. Again the main focus is upon England, although important similarities and differences with Scotland, Wales and Northern Ireland are discussed (see Box 6.1).

The nature of the voluntary sector

Historical context

Organized voluntarism expanded in the Victorian period in response to the dislocation caused by industrialization and urbanization. This is exemplified by the rise of philanthropy, civic improvement, self-help and good works (Briggs, 1959). In the health field, for example, associations emerged providing practical information about health and hygiene, alongside health services and support to the poor and sick (for instance, the Ladies' Sanitary Association of Manchester and Salford, which pioneered health visiting). Some voluntary organizations engaged in advocacy to achieve legislative ends with regard to sanitation (see, for example, Hollis, 1974). The conventional view is that the growth in state health responsibilities and functions in the twentieth century displaced the voluntary sector. However, this is an oversimplified view (Harris, 2010; Alcock, 2011; Hilton and McKay, 2011). Instead, as Lewis (1999) observed, the relationship between the state and the voluntary sector shifted, reflecting the changing roles of voluntary organizations.

They were regarded as the main providers of services (nineteenth century), complementary providers (first part of the twentieth century) and supplementary providers (latter part of the twentieth century). Their contribution and importance did not therefore decline but flourished in the substantial gaps between statutory services, especially where the state was unable or unwilling to provide services (examples include hospice care, addiction services and family planning services). The vitality of the voluntary sector under the welfare state was illustrated by the growth in new charitable registrations, which doubled between 1960 and 1980 (Alcock, 2011).

Diversity and definitions

The voluntary sector is extremely diverse (Kendall and Knapp, 1995). It contains organizations of different shapes and sizes: from organizations with multimillion pound budgets, thousands of members, supporters and volunteers, and hundreds of employees (such as the Red Cross, Macmillan Cancer Support and the British Heart Foundation), to those that are tiny. It harbours many different types of organization (hierarchical, federal and autonomous; national and local; formal and informal). Voluntary organizations can take one of several legal forms (including company limited by guarantee, charitable trust, unincorporated association, industrial and provident society, and charitable incorporated organization). Some have charitable status, while others do not. The voluntary sector covers many policy areas, including the environment, housing, sport and leisure, education, animal welfare, poverty and disadvantage, faith and religion, social support, addictions, children and young people, older people, ethnic minorities and health and social care.

The basis of most definitions of the voluntary sector lies in its 'non-profit' status (to distinguish it from business organizations), its 'non-governmental', 'autonomous' and 'voluntary' status (to distinguish it from the state sector) and its degree of organization (to distinguish it from the family, social networks or social movements). Taking this approach, Salamon and Anheier (1997) identified five core characteristics of non-profit organizations:

- Organized (possessing organizational and institutional reality)
- Private (institutionally separate from government and the public sector)
- Non-profit-distributing (do not return a profit to owners)
- Self-governing (equipped to control their own activities)
- Voluntary (non-compulsory in nature and with some degree of voluntary input).

Unsurprisingly, given the diversity of the sector, the 'labels' used to describe it are contested and reflect different perspectives (Kendall, 2009; Alcock, 2010). As Newman and Clarke (2009) observed, there is a fundamental ambiguity about voluntary organizations. These can be an instrument of the state, but can operate as autonomous sites of resistance to government and mobilize counterreaction. The terminology of the voluntary sector has shifted over time, reflecting the dominance of particular ideas (Alcock, 2010). Formerly, the terms most commonly used to describe the sector were 'the charitable sector' or 'not-for-profit' sector.

Then 'the voluntary sector' became fashionable, followed by 'the voluntary and community sector' (to reflect the informal nature of much voluntary activity). Under New Labour, the term 'third sector' was in vogue, defined officially as 'non-governmental organizations that are value-driven and which principally reinvest their surpluses to further social, environmental or cultural objectives' (Cm 7189, 2007, p. 5). The third sector included organizations such as social enterprises, cooperatives and mutuals that made a profit or surplus but allocated most of this to social objectives. In a more recent shift, the Cameron Coalition government has preferred the term 'civil society sector'. This is an even broader term that includes charitable, voluntary, community and third sector organizations along with community action and volunteering, consistent with the government's notion of a Big Society (see Box 5.2). The use of these various labels is confusing and, for the purpose of this book, except where a particular concept is being specifically addressed or discussed, the term 'voluntary sector' will be used.

Size and scope

Definitions are important, not least because they affect estimates of the size and scope of the voluntary sector. If one takes the third sector as a broad basis for calculations, the UK has 900,000 organizations (including charities, housing associations, social enterprises, mutuals, cooperatives, research organizations and non-profit-making bodies; Clark et al., 2010). In England and Wales alone, there are over 160,000 general registered charities, 60,000 social enterprises (discussed in more detail in Box 7.1), and an estimated 600,000 informal community organizations. The UK third sector had a combined income in 2009–10 of £157 billion (over 10 per cent of the gross domestic product), and combined assets of £244 billion (Clark et al., 2010). Its workforce in 2011 stood at over 765,000 people (617,000 full-time equivalents) – 2.7 per cent of the total workforce (Clark et al., 2011). In addition, around two-fifths of adults in England undertake voluntary work at least once a year (DCLG, 2011b). The majority of adults donate to charities, and over half do so in a typical month (Charities Aid Foundation and NCVO, 2010) with donations (including legacies) totalling over £12 billion for the financial year 2009/10.

   Health and social welfare is a primary focus for many voluntary organizations. One survey found that over a quarter of third sector bodies worked in the field of health and well-being (Ipsos MORI, 2011). Another found that 57 per cent of third sector employees are engaged in health and social work – the majority in social work or residential care (Clark et al., 2011). In 2007, it was estimated that 35,000 third sector organizations provided health or social care, and a further 1,600 planned to do so in the next three to five years (IFF Research, 2007). The total funding for these services was estimated at £12 billion (then 14 per cent of the health and social care budget for England). A substantial proportion of this, over £3 billion, is provided by the public sector (Curry et al., 2011). Although it was found that the vast majority of these organizations provided social care, or a mix of health and social care (IFF Research, 2007), health and well-being appears to be an area of growing interest (see Box 6.2 later in the chapter). Voluntary organizations have been active in mental health, addictions, nutrition and diet, exercise and physical activity, smoking cessation, the health of children and young people, and sexual health. Others have a bearing on health and well-being through their work in areas such as culture, equalities and civil rights, community development, social cohesion, housing, the environment and poverty relief. In addition, some contribute to the public health agenda by working with particular groups such as older people, children, young people and families, carers, ethnic minorities and faith communities. Even where voluntary organizations are not focused on specific health issues, they may be involved in prevention, signposting services and providing advocacy and support, in ways that enhance public health strategies and programmes (Curry et al., 2011; Richmond Council for Voluntary Services, 2011).

The contribution of voluntary organizations

In general, voluntary organizations are credited with advantages and strengths (see, for example, Kelly, 2007; Select Committee on Public Administration, 2008b; Martikke and Moxham, 2010; Hogg and Baines, 2011). These include:

- identifying needs and providing a better quality of services, being more responsive to the needs of service users;
- contribution to pluralism of supply, and thereby competition;
- improving efficiency (through competition, reducing bureaucracy and reducing costs through the use of lower paid workers and volunteers);
- enabling greater voice and choice for users on policy and service development, and advocating on their behalf;
- empowering users, enabling them to exert influence over professionals and take more control and responsibility for their own lives;
- building and harnessing social capital, and mobilizing financial and human resources;
- promoting community development and social cohesion;
- promoting innovation in service provision;
- bringing specialist knowledge and expertise to bear on the problem;
- filling the gaps in services left by statutory services;
- acting as a force for service integration across traditional agency boundaries.

One reason why the voluntary sector has attracted positive attention from policy-makers, especially in recent years, lies in a broad consensus about its merits and how these should be promoted. These merits have not gone totally unchallenged, however (Hogg and Baines, 2011). Some have questioned the assumption that innovation is a defining characteristic of voluntary and non-profit organizations (Osborne and Flynn, 1997; Osborne et al., 2008). Others have doubted whether the voluntary sector does actually have more specialist knowledge and expertise than other sectors, and its supposedly unique 'user focus' has also been questioned (Select Committee on Public Administration, 2008b). Questions have also been raised about the relative cost-effectiveness of the voluntary sector (see Lewis, 1999; Select Committee on Public Administration, 2011) and the benefits of pluralism and competition in public services (Kelly, 2007). As we shall see later, bringing the voluntary sector into a much more formal relationship with government may also undermine its essential qualities.

Policy on the voluntary sector

The postwar period

The voluntary sector was increasingly acknowledged by government in the postwar period. During the 1960s and 1970s, local authorities and other agencies were encouraged to work more closely with it in areas such as health, social care, housing and welfare (Deakin and Davis Smith, 2011). The government responded positively to the report of the Wolfenden Committee (Committee on Voluntary Organizations, 1978), which urged greater collaboration between statutory and voluntary sectors and emphasized the need for a long-term strategy.

The Thatcher and Major governments

The Thatcher and Major governments initiated some changes beneficial to the voluntary sector, such as amendments to charity regulation and tax rules. The Major government introduced a national volunteering programme and established the National Lottery, which raised additional funds for good causes and charities. Both governments endorsed the voluntary sector as part of their aim to strengthen individual responsibility, reduce dependence on the state and extend pluralism in public service provision. A strategic approach was, however, lacking (Kendall and Knapp, 1995). There was a strong focus on enhancing the contribution of the voluntary sector to public service provision (Home Office, 1990; Knight, 1993), although this was criticized for neglecting the important civic advocacy role of voluntary organizations (Lewis, 1999). A landmark report by the Deakin Commission (Commission on the Future of the Voluntary Sector, 1996) reiterated the civic role of voluntary organizations while echoing Wolfenden's call for a more strategic and collaborative approach. It acknowledged that voluntary organizations should become more involved in service provision, but within a clear and explicit framework. One of Deakin's key recommendations was an overarching agreement or 'concordat' between the government and the voluntary sector. Others included: clarification of the legal definition and regulation of charities; a strengthened single coherent source of expertise related to the voluntary sector in Whitehall, with a cross-government brief to raise the profile and standing of the sector and increase its contribution; closer relationships between business and the voluntary sector based on common goals; and that the independence of the voluntary sector must be recognized by all funders.

New Labour

New Labour's endorsement of communitarian ideas (Etzioni, 1993; Tam, 1998), and its support for a Third Way approach between market and state, strengthened its focus on the voluntary sector. Before coming to office, New Labour established a review of the sector (Labour Party, 1997). It responded positively to Deakin's recommendations and pledged to review charity law, establish a Compact (similar to the 'concordat' recommended by Deakin), strengthen cross-departmental cooperation within government, build closer working relationships between the voluntary and private sectors, and preserve the independence of the voluntary sector. It also endorsed explicit standards of service, and a fairer and more effective funding regime. The overarching theme was to proactively mainstream the voluntary sector and build stronger partnerships with it (Sullivan and Skelcher, 2002; Hogg and Baines, 2011), captured in Kendall's (2009) phrase, 'hyperactive mainstreaming'.

As already noted, New Labour widened the concept of the voluntary sector by endorsing social enterprises and other bodies. Furthermore, a major review of charity law was undertaken (Cabinet Office, 2002), leading to the Charities Act 2006, which redefined charity in terms of public benefit and reformulated charitable purposes. The Charity Commission, which regulates and advises charities, was reconstituted as an independent statutory body, alongside a new appeals process. The regulatory regime for charities was simplified to ease the burden on smaller organizations. A new legal form was established for charities wishing to become incorporated and limit their liability – the Charitable Incorporated Organization. Following concerns about undue restrictions on charity campaigns and lobbying (Kennedy, 2007), the Charity Commission (2008) issued guidance to clarify the legitimacy of such activities, with a proviso that charities must not undertake political activity as an end in itself. Party political activity (for example, support for party candidates in elections), remained out of bounds.

Labour also reorganized existing central government structures that managed relationships with the voluntary sector (Alcock, 2011). An Active Community Unit was established in the Home Office in 1999. A Civil Renewal Unit was later created to promote citizenship and community action. Subsequently, in 2003, both the Civil Renewal Unit and the Active Community Unit (and a separate unit dealing with charities) were brought together in an Active Communities Directorate of the Home Office. In 2006, the Active Communities Directorate was merged with a Social Enterprise Unit (established in 2001 in the Department of Trade and Industry) to create an Office of the Third Sector (OTS), based in the Cabinet Office. Although the search for a rational structure within government to promote and develop the third sector was welcomed, such constant reorganization was confusing and destabilizing (Zimmeck et al., 2011).

The Compact

The Compact on Relations between Government and the Voluntary and Community Sector in England (Cm 4100, 1998; hereafter referred to as 'the Compact') outlined shared principles (such as 'voluntary action is an essential component of a democratic society'). It also set out undertakings by government (including 'to recognize and support the independence of the sector', 'to develop in consultation with the sector a code of good practice to address principles of good funding for government departments', 'to appraise new policies and procedures, particularly at the developmental stage, so as to identify as far as possible implications for the sector', and 'to consult the sector on issues that are likely to affect it'), and undertakings by the voluntary sector (such as 'to maintain high standards of governance and conduct', 'to respect the confidentiality of government information', and 'to involve users wherever possible in the development and management of activities and services'). The Compact included provisions for a joint annual review, and a process for resolving disagreements and complaints.

Separate national compacts were introduced in Scotland, Wales and Northern Ireland, which developed their own policies on the voluntary sector (Morison, 2000; Box 6.1). Local areas were encouraged to formulate their own compacts as well. A number of good practice guides on key issues (volunteering, consultation, black and ethnic minority groups, funding and community groups) were later produced to supplement the Compact. A 'refreshed' Compact was launched in 2009, which included new commitments from both the government and the voluntary sector, notably with regard to equal opportunities (CompactVoice et al., 2009). Following the change of government in 2010, the Compact was again revised, discussed further below in the context of the Coalition's policies on the voluntary sector.

Box 6.1	The voluntary sector in Scotland, Wales and Northern Ireland

Although the advent of devolution in the UK created important new space for policy development in the third sector, the direction of travel in all four regimes has been remarkably similar (Alcock, 2012). For example, each part of the UK introduced its own Compacts between the government and the voluntary sector, established similar institutions within government to promote the sector, and adopted schemes to build capacity and develop the voluntary sector as a service provider. Scotland and Northern Ireland, like England and Wales, also embarked on reform of their charity laws. But despite the similarities, there are also important differences between the countries of the UK.

In Scotland, the voluntary sector is more generously funded by the state than it is in England, and receives more funds through local government. There are some institutional differences, too, with the creation of Third Sector Interfaces between the third sector and local government. In relation to health, the Scottish voluntary sector has been acknowledged as a key partner in official reports and policy documents (see, for example, Kerr, 2005; Scottish Government, 2007a). A national body represents voluntary health organizations (Voluntary Health Scotland [VHS], established in 2000). Compared with the nearest equivalent English body, National Voices, VHS appears to have a wider remit, covering health and well-being issues as well as care, support and treatment. The Scottish voluntary sector also operates in a different health service structure from that of England. Voluntary organizations are included in Community Health Partnerships (CHPs; to be replaced by Health and Social Care Partnerships; see Chapter 3). These interact with local authorities, health boards and other partnership bodies, such as the Community Planning Partnerships, which have a remit for promoting health and well-being and reducing health inequalities. Although there is evidence to suggest that CHPs and other health and social care bodies have made efforts to involve the voluntary sector, there is considerable room for improvement (Ball et al., 2010; Watt et al., 2010). VHS has issued guidance to CHPs on involving the sector (Voluntary Health Scotland, 2005, 2007) but remains dissatisfied. Indeed, its own research into voluntary sector experiences of engagement with statutory bodies (Voluntary Health Scotland, 2009a, 2009b, 2011) found persistent problems, including a lack of funding for participation and representation, a lack of influence over strategy, and a failure to utilize the voluntary sector fully in service development.

In Wales, as in Scotland, the voluntary sector receives a greater proportion of its funds from the state than in England (Alcock, 2012). Moreover, there is a specific statutory duty placed on the Welsh government to promote the interests of voluntary organizations. This requires it to adopt a scheme to provide assistance (financial and other means of support) to voluntary organizations and consult them when exercising its functions. Wales has a Third Sector Partnership Council, chaired by a minister. In addition to the Compact for Wales, there is a Strategic Action Plan for the voluntary sector (Welsh Assembly Government, 2008). Some argue that Wales has had the advantage of a strong voluntary sector infrastructure at local level (through the Welsh Council for Voluntary Action networks and local intermediary bodies; Green and Drakeford, 2001).

Like their Scottish counterparts, Welsh voluntary organizations appear to have a stronger focus on health and well-being issues compared with England. This perspective is encouraged by the Welsh government. In addition to the national funding scheme for voluntary organizations, there is a health promotion voluntary grant scheme. Funds have been allocated to a range of projects including the prevention of accidents and injuries in children, the promotion of 'green gyms' (which encourage people to exercise outdoors, for example by working on conservation projects) and the prevention of self-harm. Local authorities and local health boards must consult with voluntary organizations (and other stakeholders) when devising health, social care and well-being plans for their area. Local health boards are required to have a member drawn from the voluntary sector. There are also opportunities to influence the local public health agenda through health, social care and well-being alliances (some of which have been renamed as health and well-being partnerships), which bring together local agencies, voluntary groups and other stakeholders to discuss priorities and develop action plans. Voluntary groups also seek to influence the community strategies of local authorities, which have implications for health, well-being and social care. Furthermore, voluntary organizations in Wales have been actively involved in specific public health initiatives and health-related programmes in areas such as sexual health, mental health, accident prevention and Sure Start.

Northern Ireland developed a very distinctive approach to the voluntary sector (Acheson, 1989; Kearney and Williamson, 2001; Alcock, 2012). This arose from the 'troubles' and associated sectarian divide and the failure of local government to address the needs of all people in the Province. This meant that voluntary organizations had a key role in meeting needs, combatting discrimination, building social capital and providing a voice for those not represented in the political process. They were supported by central government. Funding for the sector tended to bypass local government, going directly to the voluntary organizations themselves. Voluntary organizations in Northern Ireland still receive the highest levels of state funding in the UK relative to their total income, and the vast majority of this comes via central/national government. They have also generated significant funds from the European Union, much specifically linked to building peace in the Province, although this has been reduced significantly in recent years (Alcock, 2012). Local government has played a relatively small role in the development of the voluntary sector in Northern Ireland compared with other parts of the UK. However, this is starting to change with the resumption of devolved government (in 2007) and local government reform.

The voluntary sector has actively participated in health policy and service development in Northern Ireland. Public health strategies have emphasized the importance of the voluntary sector in partnership working, especially with regard to social, economic and environmental causes of illness, health inequalities and specific health issues such as alcohol, obesity, smoking and accident prevention. Northern Ireland's Health Promotion Agency encouraged the formation of health alliances, including the voluntary sector. In addition, public health strategies, programmes such as Health Action Zones and Healthy Living Centres, local Health Improvement Plans and 'Investing for Health' local partnerships, included and involved voluntary organizations (DHSSNI, 1997; DHSSPS, 2002, 2004).

The Compact had an important symbolic effect and was seen in a positive light by the voluntary sector (Lewis, 2005). Its main contribution perhaps was to give a 'feelgood factor' to relations between the statutory and voluntary sectors (Zimmeck et al., 2011; NAO, 2012). But there were shortcomings in its implementation, to some extent due to its lack of legal force. Consequently, new bodies were established to strengthen implementation: the Commission on the Compact (to oversee implementation and promote good practice); Compact Voice (to coordinate and promote the views of the sector about the Compact, and to provide practical help, training and guidance and share best practice); and Compact Advocacy (to help with complaints about breaches of the Compact). However, this created a confusing institutional context (since rationalized by the Coalition government). The lack of clarity between the remits of these bodies was noted in an evaluation of the Compact (Zimmeck et al., 2011), which found other shortcomings in implementation, such as poor leadership and insufficient administrative support, weaknesses in the mechanisms for liaison between the government and the sector, lack of resources and legitimacy (in the case of Compact Voice) and a lack of independence from government (in the case of the Commission on the Compact).

The Compact was largely ineffective in promoting the voluntary sector as an equal partner in policy-making (HM Treasury, 2002; Roberts, 2008; Alcock, 2011). Scepticism was reflected in relatively low levels of satisfaction among voluntary organizations about their ability to influence decisions (see Ipsos MORI, 2011). There were difficulties, however, in measuring the effect of engagement with the sector, due to a lack of comprehensive data about consultation processes and the roles of voluntary organizations in relation to them (Zimmeck et al., 2011). Nonetheless, New Labour continued to place great emphasis on building effective long-term relationships with the sector (HM Treasury, 2002; Cm 7189, 2007). Efforts were made to strengthen advisory and consultative processes by funding strategic partners (providing grants to voluntary organizations seen as able to represent the wider sector) and by rationalizing existing advisory bodies. Central government Public Service Agreements emphasized the importance of the voluntary sector and active communities. Local performance measures and indicators were introduced to reflect this priority (HM Government, 2007a). Efforts were also made to improve funding systems and voluntary sector capacity.

Funding, capacity and contracts

Funding has been the most common area of complaint under the Compact (NAO, 2012). This reflects Zimmeck et al.'s (2011) findings that the provisions on funding and procurement had been halting and uneven. Related to this, capacity has been another key issue. Following a report on voluntary sector funding by the Better Regulation Task Force (1998) and a cross-cutting review of the third sector (HM Treasury, 2002), greater efforts were made to strengthen capacity (Home Office, 2004). New funding schemes were introduced: Futurebuilders, which gave third sector bodies access to loan capital; and ChangeUp (and from 2006, Capacitybuilders), which enabled investment in infrastructure. These schemes were found to have delivered some benefits to the voluntary sector, with frontline organizations now receiving better coordinated and more effective support services and being in a better position to win contracts (NAO, 2009). However, weaknesses in programme management and in demonstrating value for money were also evident.

A further development was the National Commissioning Programme, which sought to expand opportunities for voluntary organizations and other third sector bodies to deliver services on behalf of the state (Office of the Third Sector 2006; Audit Commission, 2007b). It aimed to deliver training for commissioners on the benefits of the voluntary sector, to provide greater opportunities for voluntary organizations to shape the delivery of public services, to ensure that commissioning met the needs of users, carers and communities, and to strengthen the ability of voluntary organizations to secure contracts to deliver services. A skills strategy was also proposed (although this was slow to develop; see Wilkes, 2010). As a result of these initiatives, the dependence of voluntary organizations on state funding increased. The statutory funding of charities increased substantially after 2000–01, from £8.4 billion to £12 billion in 2006–07 (Kane et al., 2009, cited by Macmillan, 2010). Furthermore, income from contracts became more important. Between 2000 and 2007, grant-based funding slightly declined while income from contracts more than doubled (calculated from Kane et al., 2009, cited by Alcock, 2011). Statutory funding represents more than a third of voluntary sector income in total, although only one in four organizations actually receives funding from state sources (Macmillan, 2010).

Greater dependence on state funding raised fears that the independence and autonomy of the voluntary sector would be undermined (Kelly, 2007; Carmel and Harlock, 2008; Select Committee on Public Administration, 2008b, 2011; Martikke and Moxham 2010). There are obvious tensions between service provider and advocacy roles (Lewis, 2005). The state's superior resources and political power could force voluntary organizations to conform to a top-down agenda (Hodgson, 2004; Independence Panel, 2012). The emphasis on commissioning and contracting may further bind voluntary organizations to public sector processes and centrally set standards of performance and delivery (Carmel and Harlock, 2008). These concerns have some foundation (Martikke and Moxham, 2010), although the evidence so far is mixed (Macmillan, 2010). Furthermore, as the Select Committee on Public Administration (2008b) observed, as long as voluntary and third sector involvement in public services remains at a low level, many of the risks are perhaps exaggerated. Nonetheless, there should be no complacency, and it is certainly an area where more primary research is required.

Contracting seems to favour larger voluntary organizations and social enterprises, which have greater capacity to bid than smaller organizations (Select Committee on Public Administration, 2011). It also tends to favour the private sector, given its greater experience and resources, and there are additional dangers that voluntary organizations could become mere subcontractors, considerably weakening their position. There is plenty of evidence that processes of contracting operate against the interests of the voluntary sector (Cairns et al., 2006; NAO, 2007). Commissioners have a poor understanding of the sector and its added value (Aldridge, 2005; Audit Commission, 2007b; Select Committee on Public Administration, 2008b; Jackson, 2010). There has sometimes been a lack of trust and poor communication in the relationship between local commissioning bodies and the voluntary sector (Jackson, 2010). Voluntary organizations have had limited opportunities to be involved in service design (Martikke and Moxham, 2010). Short-term contracts (often annual contracts) have prevailed, inhibiting service development and longer term planning. Even larger charities have faced difficulties in dealing with multiple, complex funding regimes (NAO, 2007). Commissioners have also been reluctant to reimburse the full costs of service delivery (including overheads) borne by the sector (NAO, 2005). Although government has acknowledged these problems and sought to prevent them, such practices have persisted.

The local level

Local authorities (and other public agencies) were expected to include voluntary organizations in their engagement processes. As noted, local authorities were encouraged to establish local compacts, and most did so (Craig et al., 2002). Zimmeck et al. (2011) observed a variation in the content, longevity and impact of local compacts, noting that the best local compacts made significant and valuable contributions to improving relationships. Beyond this, voluntary bodies were included on the local implementation bodies of major programmes such as housing and regeneration. They were consulted by local government on their community plans, although this involvement was described by one study as 'incredibly limited' (ODPM, 2005). The same study found that few community strategies referred to the local compact.

Meanwhile, Local Strategic Partnerships (LSPs; see Chapter 3) were expected to fully involve voluntary sector representatives in developing and coordinating strategies (Taylor, 2006). It was found that over nine out of 10 LSPs had voluntary sector representatives (DCLG, 2009; NAVCA, 2011). However, problems arose in practice. For example, Marks (2007), in a study of the involvement of voluntary organizations in partnerships tackling health inequalities, found significant barriers and tensions that prevented them from playing a full role in the development of local strategies. Furthermore, other research revealed that voluntary groups were stretched and underresourced, and that infrastructure and resources were needed to ensure that LSPs engaged effectively with voluntary groups and the wider community (ODPM, 2006; see also Russell, 2005). The ODPM study found a wide variation in patterns of voluntary representation (particularly with regard to the types of organization involved, the level of representation and the means of selection). Although the voluntary sector was represented on most LSPs, they often felt like junior partners and lacked influence. Time and resources constrained voluntary sector involvement in LSPs. The culture of partnership working was also important. Another key factor was uncertainty and confusion about the role of the voluntary sector in relation to LSPs (a point also made by Marks, 2007). Capacity-building was identified as a prerequisite for full participation of the voluntary sector as equals.

These concerns were echoed by a further report (DCLG, 2011a), which urged clarification of the voluntary sector role in LSPs. This study found that voluntary sector partners were less satisfied than other stakeholders with engagement in LSPs. Particular tensions were identified between the need to be inclusive and the impera-tive to devise arrangements that were streamlined and action-oriented. However, the report acknowledged that LSPs did provide an entry point to strategic decision-making for the voluntary sector and opportunities for working in partnership on key thematic areas. The Audit Commission (2009), meanwhile, urged that more be done to encourage participation from the voluntary sector, including more resources and improvements in modes of engagement. This was echoed by the Strategic Review of Health Inequalities in England (2010), which called for LSPs to engage the voluntary sector in a systematic way to maximize the potential for participation, empowerment and capacity-building. In contrast, the National Association for Voluntary and Community Action (NAVCA; 2011) indicated broadly positive views from voluntary sector representatives about their current role on LSPs. It maintained that representation on LSPs allowed the voice of disengaged people to be heard, enabled community involvement in decision-making, ensured activity was relevant to local needs, and conveyed the voluntary sector perspective on service design and delivery. The NAVCA report also found evidence that the influence of the voluntary sector was significantly higher where it was represented on LSPs.

Difficulties in the relationship between the voluntary sector and local partner-ship bodies reflected wider problems of engagement. These included raised expec-tations that could be met by public bodies. Involvement in deliberations about policy and service development does not guarantee influence (Baggott et al., 2005). There is often a danger of 'tokenism' (see Chapter 5), where public bodies simply go through the motions of engaging with the sector without genuinely seeking to incorporate its views. A further problem is that engagement imposes costs on the voluntary sector. Organizations are often approached by a number of public bodies, even on similar issues (and occasionally by different parts of the same body on the same issue). This places a burden on voluntary bodies and leading to them becoming overstretched and experiencing 'consultation fatigue' (see Chapter 5). This can be addressed to some extent by better coordination among public bodies when engaging with the voluntary sector.

Another commonly identified problem lies in the representative role of voluntary groups. This is problematic because, for practical reasons, not all groups can be directly represented on advisory, consultative and decision-making bodies. As the sector is diverse, it is impossible for one group to speak on behalf of the whole sector (ODPM, 2006). Umbrella bodies and alliances are perhaps able to speak with some legitimacy, but even they have difficulty speaking for the sector as a whole. A related danger is that the same individuals can become identified as the voice of the sector, often labelled 'the usual suspects' (see Chapter 5). Added to this is the difficulty of securing involvement from some organizations, particularly those which are small, poorly resourced or lack capacity, and which speak for people and communities that are hard to reach. Although engagement with the voluntary sector has been seen as good practice to enable greater community participation in policy and decisions about services, it is not unproblematic and, if undertaken in ignorance of the pitfalls, can be not only a waste of time and resources, but also a gross misrepresentation of the views of voluntary service providers, service users and the wider public.

The Coalition government and the voluntary sector

Adopting the rhetoric of the 'Big Society' (see Box 5.2), the Cameron government emphasized the role of voluntary groups in civil society and in public services (Cabinet Office, 2010). It sought to redefine the voluntary sector and third sector as Civil Society Organizations. An Office for Civil Society (OCS) replaced the OTS within the Cabinet Office. However, despite the government's declared aim of raising the profile of civil society, the minister heading the OCS was appointed at a lower rank than the Labour government's minister for the third sector.

The Coalition revised the national Compact, making it clear that all departments must include it in their business plans. The new Compact (HM Government, 2010b) was intended as a more easily understood and practical document that would strengthen accountability and align the Compact with the 'Big Society'. It set out commitments for government and the Civil Society Organizations under several key 'outcomes': a strong, diverse and independent society; effective and transparent design and development of policies, programmes and public services; responsive and high-quality programmes and services; clear arrangements for managing changes to programmes and services; and an equal and fair society. Key commitments of the previous Compacts were retained, and there were additional ones, for example a reduction in government bureaucracy (something which the previous government had pledged following a critical report from the Better Regulation Task Force, 2005). Other new commitments included to improve commissioning, to take into account social, environmental and economic value in policies and programmes, and to strengthen accountability in relation to the implementation of the Compact. However, the new Compact was shorter than the previous versions and much less detailed. Some observers also detected significant nuances (Zimmeck et al., 2011). Unlike the original Compact, it was not a command paper. The new Compact focused more strongly on public service delivery and placed greater emphasis on commitments and outcomes rather than shared values and principles.

The National Audit Office (NAO; 2012) undertook an analysis of the implementation of the 2010 Compact. While endorsing it as a framework for shaping partnership and strengthening accountability, the NAO found several shortcomings. It urged a stronger approach to improve leadership, strengthen monitoring and facilitate the sharing of good practice. It found that the 12-week 'benchmark' for consulting the sector on policy was often not met. It discovered that information about non-compliance with the Compact was not centrally analysed, and that departments lacked arrangements to assure compliance (despite being required to report this in their business plans). The NAO also found that the role of the OCS in relation to the Compact was unclear. It called for a more systematic approach on the part of departments (and especially the OCS) in monitoring and reporting, and clearer responsibilities within government to oversee implementation and promote good practice. This was echoed by a further investigation (Elkins, 2012), which found that government departments were failing to record and/or retrieve information about their compliance with the Compact. It discovered that no system had been introduced across central government to ensure that commitments under the Compact were being effectively monitored. This report called for government departments to collate and publish information about compliance with the Compact, on engagement with the voluntary sector and on funding. It recommended that departments report on voluntary sector contracting and subcontracting to ensure that the Compact's principles were being applied in practice. The report also called on the Cabinet Office to publish a progress report on the implementation of the Compact.

The Coalition government also abolished a number of institutional arrangements. The Commission on the Compact was abolished, and its role in monitoring implementation was passed to Compact Voice and the OCS, a move criticized for weakening monitoring and accountability. In addition, the Capacity-builders programme was brought to an end. A key advisory body that had served as a channel of advice and communication between the sector and the OTS was abolished. Furthermore, the Strategic Partners programme, which provided support for key voluntary organizations enabling them to provide a voice for the sector at national level, suffered a drastic reduction in its funding, which was planned to cease entirely in 2014. These moves were criticized for undermining the position of the voluntary sector.

Furthermore, planned public sector funding cuts looked set to hit voluntary organizations hard (NEF, 2010; ACEVO, 2011; Pattie and Johnston, 2011; Select Committee on Public Administration, 2011; Independence Panel, 2012). OCS spending on voluntary organizations was due to fall by 61 per cent in three years. Further cuts were inevitable as NHS and local government budgets came under pressure due to efficiency savings and cuts (ACEVO, 2011). A comprehensive analysis of the impact of budget cuts found that the voluntary sector expected to lose £2.8 billion in state support between 2012–13 and 2015–16 (Kane and Allen, 2011). However, this report pointed out that cuts would be felt unevenly across the sectors as different parts of government and programmes were not uniformly affected. Indeed, some budgets (notably in the health arena) were likely to receive increased resources. It also found that over half of local authorities were disproportionately cutting voluntary sector budgets (that is, by more than average). Moreover, it found that some local authorities were not making strategic long-term decisions, and that this was damaging to the voluntary sector and communities.

On a more positive note, plans for a Big Society Bank (now renamed Big Society Capital) were finalized, with £600 million capital (the majority from dormant bank accounts and the rest from banks) to invest in social enterprises. The fund is seeking to attract further private investment, although it is difficult to see where this will come from in an era of persistent economic stagnation. There have been concerns about the relatively small size of this fund and delays in establishing it (Select Committee on Public Administration, 2011). In another initiative, the government increased incentives for people to bequeath money to charities and made it easier for charities to claim tax relief from donations. However, contradictory plans in the 2012 Budget to limit tax relief for the richest donors angered charities, and the government was forced to backtrack. Meanwhile, responsibility for the National Lottery's Big Lottery Fund was transferred from the Department of Culture Media and Sport to the Cabinet Office. The Fund launched a new £20 million 'Building Capabilities for Impact and Legacy' programme to support capacity-building in the voluntary sector. New directives meanwhile required the Fund to focus more on supporting and empowering communities. A Transition Fund was also introduced to help voluntary organizations facing financial problems, although this was extremely limited (Select Committee on Public Administration, 2011). In addition, new funding schemes were introduced to support voluntary and community groups at local level (Community First and Transforming Local Infrastructure).

Other Coalition policies had important implications for the voluntary sector. A commitment to opening up public services to the voluntary and private sectors could potentially lead to an expansion in both (Cm 8145, 2011). To address some of the problems experienced with contracting in the past, discussed above, a consultation on modernizing commissioning was undertaken. The government's plans to give local communities more power over decision-making (see Chapter 4) also had implications for the voluntary and community sector, potentially increasing opportunities for it to engage more in local decision-making and service provision. In addition, the government piloted community budgets, which involved local voluntary groups and the wider public in debates about local spending priorities. Meanwhile changes in existing local processes (such as abolishing Local Area Agreements and Comprehensive Area Assessment, and allowing local areas to be more flexible in how they determine priorities and partnership working arrangements) have implications for the way in which the voluntary sector interacts with local governance structures. It could destabilize voluntary sector partnerships with local agencies, although it is possible that new and possibly more productive partnerships could be formed at the community level, if indeed power and responsibility are devolved as promised.

The voluntary sector and health

The contribution of the voluntary sector

As noted earlier in this chapter, health and well-being is an important area of work for the voluntary sector. The contribution of the voluntary sector to health can be outlined as follows (WHO, 2001; Wanless, 2004; Cm 7432, 2008; ACEVO, 2010; Strategic Review of Health Inequalities in England, 2010; Curry et al., 2011; House of Lords Select Committee on Science and Technology, 2011). Voluntary organizations can:

- help prevent disease and promote health by providing information to their members and the wider public;
- promote self-help and self care;
- gather information from the community about health needs, health trends and threats to health;
- contribute to planning and service delivery, ensuring that user and public perspectives are fed into decision-making;
- campaign and lobby on health issues;
- give voice to marginalized and disadvantaged groups;
- help identify and overcome barriers to disease prevention and health promotion (such as social attitudes, cultural norms and economic disincentives);
- help integrate services (by interacting with multiple agencies that have specific responsibilities and functions that affect health and well-being);
- develop and provide services that are more flexible and suited to users' needs;
- harness and mobilize community resources and assets, including volunteers;
- link into wider voluntary sector networks that can help promote health;
- raise funds for, facilitate and undertake research.

Policies on the voluntary health sector

The importance of working with voluntary organizations on health and welfare matters was the subject of Ministry of Health guidance in the 1960s (Deakin and Davis Smith, 2011). Later, the government took powers to fund voluntary agencies in this field (Section 64 of the Health Services and Public Health Act 1968) and empowered local authorities to make grants to voluntary organizations and assist them in other ways (such as the provision of support services and equipment). In the 1970s, the voluntary sector was represented on the newly established Community Health Councils (CHCs; see Chapter 5). CHCs worked alongside voluntary organizations on issues of common interest at local level, and at national level (via the Association of Community Health Councils in England and Wales). The role of the voluntary sector was acknowledged in specific policies, particularly in the field of community care. This continued throughout the 1980s, with health authorities expected to consult with the voluntary sector (DHSS, 1981). In 1985, voluntary organizations were allocated a place on Joint Consultative Committees, which advised the NHS and local authorities on the planning and funding of services at the interface of health and social care, and other areas of joint significance. In the late 1980s, the NHS was urged to work more closely with the voluntary sector specifically in relation to public health (Cm 289, 1988).

The emphasis on working with the voluntary health sector continued throughout the 1990s, and there were three main drivers. First, the introduction of the commissioning within the NHS offered more opportunities for voluntary organizations to become involved in the provision of services on behalf of the NHS. It also increased opportunities to get involved in the commissioning process, particularly with regard to identifying needs and representing the views of users, carers and the wider public. Second, national public health strategy (Cm 1986, 1992) acknowledged that voluntary organizations could help improve the health of the population, and identified them as key partners within 'healthy alliances'. This was followed by guidance on public health responsibilities which urged that voluntary organizations be provided with support and opportunities to contribute to local public health activities (Wyatt, 2002). Third, increasing attention paid to patient and public involvement (see Chapter 5) highlighted the importance of voluntary organizations as advocates, representatives and sources of expertise in health policy, planning and service delivery. Health authorities were expected to have a strategic plan for consulting with local stakeholders, including voluntary groups. The Patient Partnership Strategy, mentioned in Chapter 5, was developed with input from voluntary health organizations. This strategy acknowledged the potential contribution of patients' groups, umbrella organizations and local representative organizations in informing strategies and plans at national and local level.

New Labour's support for partnership

These policy trends strengthened under New Labour, further increasing opportunities for the voluntary sector to engage with the NHS. Health authorities were expected to work in partnership with the voluntary sector. NHS guidance stated that the voluntary sector should be engaged in the process of formulating local health improvement programmes and in alliances to promote health (Wyatt, 2002). The contribution of the voluntary sector to health improvement, and the need to work with it in partnership, was referred to in three key White Papers: *Saving Lives* (Cm 4386, 1999), *Choosing Health* (Cm 6374, 2004) and *Our Health, Our Care, Our Say* (Cm 6737, 2006). There was particular emphasis on the ability of voluntary organizations to identify and articulate the needs of disadvantaged communities and help address health inequalities.

The decision by New Labour to retain the division between commissioners and providers was also significant. World Class Commissioning (see Chapters 3 and 5), included standards on working with patients and the public. Voluntary organizations were seen as able to contribute to commissioning, the assessment of needs (increasingly important with the advent of Joint Strategic Needs Assessments [JSNAs]; see Chapters 3 and 4), the representation of user, carer and public perspectives, and the monitoring and evaluation of the quality of services. The government's patient choice agenda also to some extent enhanced the role of voluntary organizations. Although choice was defined in individualistic terms, the voluntary sector was able to advise on and support patient choice in relation to particular medical conditions while highlighting barriers to choice for disadvantaged and vulnerable groups in the population (Cm 6079, 2003). Furthermore, voluntary organizations acted as service facilitators, signposting services, as well as providers of services in their own right.

New Labour's policy on patient and public involvement (see Chapter 5) also had implications for the voluntary sector. The imposition of statutory duties on NHS bodies to consult with and involve the public and service users reinforced existing relationships with the voluntary sector. In 2003, CHCs (which involved and worked with voluntary organizations) were replaced by Patient and Public Involvement Forums (PPIFs), located in Primary Care Trusts and NHS Trusts. Like the CHCs, these new bodies also contained voluntary sector representatives (of patients, users and carers). Voluntary organizations also provided support services to PPIFs as 'hosts' (see Chapter 5). In 2008, PPIFs were replaced by Local Involvement Networks (LINks). These new bodies comprised local networks of individuals and organizations, including voluntary and community organizations. In a similar way to PPIFs, LINks were supported by an independent 'host' organization (usually a voluntary or third sector organization).

Following *Saving Lives* (Cm 4386, 1999), the National Forum of Non-Governmental Public Health Organizations was established to bring together national policy-makers and non-governmental organizations on matters of public health. It aimed to facilitate dialogue and provide expert advice on public health issues. Its membership, which began with around 30 organizations, expanded to over a hundred by 2009 (by which time it had become known as the NGO Forum). This included professional groups and trade unions (for example, the Royal College of Physicians and Unite) as well as voluntary health organizations and patients' groups (such as the Terrence Higgins Trust and the Patients' Association) and organizations with a broader consumer or welfare agenda (for example, Which? and Save the Children). With funding from the Department of Health (DH), the NGO Forum developed resources (such as guides for the voluntary sector on health inequalities and a regular newsletter for members and stakeholders), hosted conferences and workshops, contributed to training and development programmes, participated in Select Committee inquiries and government consultations. In 2007, an agreement was drawn up to establish principles of joint working between the DH and the NGO Forum. However, DH funding was subsequently discontinued, and it appears that currently the NGO Forum is no longer active.

Specific programmes and policies introduced by New Labour offered greater opportunities for the voluntary sector to get involved in policy-making. Policies on alcohol, tobacco, obesity and other public health issues emphasized the importance of working in alliances with voluntary organizations (see Box 6.2 later in the chapter). Moreover, cross-cutting programmes aimed at improving health and well-being, such as Health Action Zones, Healthy Living Centres, Sure Start and Communities for Health, involved partnership working that included the voluntary sector.

Under New Labour, the DH sought to build a strategic partnership with the voluntary sector, reflecting wider efforts to mainstream the sector, as discussed above. An agreement was drawn up with the aim of establishing and maintaining strategic engagement and partnership at the national and local levels (DH, 2004). It emphasized the involvement of the voluntary sector in needs assessment, planning and service provision. It recommended the inclusion of voluntary organizations on partnership bodies and closer cooperation between the NHS, local government and the voluntary sector to develop shared aims and approaches on issues such as workforce development (for example, training and skills development), capacity-building and information-sharing.

This was followed in 2006 by the establishment of a task force to help voluntary organizations bid for health and social care contracts. The task force identified barriers to the involvement of voluntary sector providers and ways of overcoming them (DH, 2006b). It also led to the dissemination of guidance to Primary Care Trusts and voluntary organizations to encourage good practice in commissioning, and to improve opportunities for the voluntary sector. In addition, an Innovation, Excellence and Service Development Fund was established as part of the government's Third Sector Investment Programme. This was aimed at stimulating innovative projects, improving partnership working, improving services and developing voluntary sector capacity. Notably, this funded projects in public health and well-being, as well as in health service and social care provision.

Acknowledgement of the voluntary sector as a key policy stakeholder was reflected in the representation of voluntary health organizations on the DH's National Stakeholder Forum (including Action on Smoking and Health, Diabetes UK and the British Heart Foundation) alongside representatives from NHS bodies, trade unions and professional associations. Furthermore, in 2009, a Strategic Partner programme was introduced, which funded national voluntary groups to build capacity within the voluntary sector for engagement in the NHS and care system, to bring the sector's expertise and voice to the national policy process, and to act as a channel of communication between the DH and the voluntary sector. The scheme was later expanded to cover 25 organizations in total (including Age UK, the Men's Health Forum and the National Heart Forum).

Coalition policy and the voluntary health sector

The White Paper *Healthy Lives, Healthy People* (Cm 7985, 2010) continued the emphasis on the role of the voluntary sector in public health and the need to work in partnership with it. The voluntary sector was seen as a crucial part of harnessing efforts across society to improve health. The White Paper acknowledged that voluntary organizations already provided services, acted as advocates (especially for disadvantaged groups) and were catalysts for action. It stated that partnership working would be encouraged, to address health challenges and offer opportunities for providers from all sectors (including the voluntary sector) to offer relevant services. It envisaged that, where appropriate, voluntary groups would be represented on the new Health and Wellbeing Boards (see Chapter 4), and would have a stronger role in JSNA and the production of Joint Health and Wellbeing Strategies (JHWSs). Guidance on the operation of JHWSs, JSNAs and Health and Wellbeing Boards did acknowledge the importance of voluntary sector input (NHS Confederation et al., 2011, 2012a; DH, 2013a). Despite pressure from the voluntary sector, however, the legislation did not guarantee a seat for voluntary organizations on Health and Wellbeing Boards (although they can be included at the discretion of the local authority or the board itself). Research into shadow Health and Wellbeing Boards found that voluntary groups were represented on over half of the boards (Humphries et al., 2012).

The Coalition government retained some of Labour's voluntary health sector programmes, notably the Strategic Partner programme and the Innovation, Excellence and Service Development programme. This reflected its view that the voluntary sector would have a much greater role in health and social care provision in the future. The Coalition's NHS reforms aimed to create greater pluralism in the supply of health services, including voluntary sector provision (Cm 7881, 2010). As noted in Chapter 4, the government was forced to dilute its proposals – while still increasing the scope for private and voluntary sectors to provide NHS-funded services. Criticism has persisted, however, with some maintaining that the role of smaller voluntary organizations in provision could actually be undermined (ACEVO, 2010; Curry et al., 2011).

Another relevant aspect of the Coalition's health policies was the reform of patient and public involvement. As shown in Chapter 5, this new system involved a new national body (Healthwatch England) and bodies at a local level (local healthwatch) to hold the NHS, public health and social care services to account, and to raise issues and concerns from the perspective of patients, users, carers and the wider public. The original intention was that local healthwatch bodies would be statutory organizations. At a late stage, the government decided that it would instead comprise social enterprises (and that certain functions could be subcontracted out to other organizations). This represented a considerable boost to this part of the third sector, but there were concerns that it would lead to fragmentation and could undermine the role of existing voluntary organizations (particularly those that had been active under previous systems of patient and public involvement). Indeed, a lack of engagement with the voluntary sector in the design and development of local healthwatch was identified in some local areas (LGA et al., 2012b). Subsequently, however, the government introduced regulations which enabled charities to be counted as social enterprises for the purpose of providing local healthwatch services, thus enabling them to continue to support patient and public involvement (see Chapter 5).

Impact on partnership working

There is very little research on the relationships between the government, public bodies and the voluntary health sector. Existing research can be analysed under two headings: studies at national level and those at local level.

National-level interaction

No systematic study has been undertaken of the relationship between national government bodies and the voluntary health sector as a whole. However, there has been some research into the relationship between government and health consumer and patients' organizations (HCPOs) (Wood, 2000; Baggott et al., 2005), an important subset of the voluntary health sector. Many HCPOs are focused on issues around information and the care, support and treatment of individual patients or groups of people with similar conditions. Some are significant service providers. Examples include Macmillan Cancer Support, Mind, Age UK, Diabetes UK, the National Childbirth Trust and the British Heart Foundation. Studies of HCPOs demonstrate that some have built close working relationships with government, receive substantial funding and are consulted on a wide range of health policy and service issues. Although many have access to government institutions and are involved in policy processes, most lack the political leverage of established interests in the health policy arena, such as the professions (in particular the medical profession) and industrial interests (principally, the drugs industry and private healthcare providers). There are wide inequalities in the HCPO sector, with a few well-resourced, well-connected and politically skilled organizations alongside many others that lack the capacity and resources to shape agendas and exert influence over decision-makers. This profile mirrors the voluntary sector as a whole.

Although the primary focus of most HCPOs is on specific health conditions and on matters of support, care and treatment for those affected, some have a broader agenda. They tend to speak on behalf of particular population groups (children, older people, men, women, ethnic groups and people with a range of disabilities). Others are alliances or umbrella groups bringing together a broader collection of interests. To address the fragmented nature of representation in this area, efforts have been made to strengthen formal alliances. For example, in 2008, National Voices was created, representing over 150 organizations, as a means of establishing a more coherent voice for patient and consumer interests in health at the national level. This body has received funds from the DH under the Strategic Partner Programme (see above). Other cross-sector groups include Network for Patients, an alliance of 30 charities established in 2009, which provides a common voice on issues affecting patients and the public.

Although HCPOs have tended to focus on individual care and treatment rather than public health issues, such as health promotion and disease prevention, there are exceptions. Breast cancer groups, for example, have campaigned for improvements in screening programmes, while some have explored environmental and public health issues in relation to the disease (Batt, 1994; Klawiter, 1999). Other HCPOs have shifted towards a more preventive focus in fields as diverse as pregnancy and infant loss (Layne, 2006) and asthma (Brown et al., 2003). In some areas, HCPOs have always had a strong prevention and public health element in their work, for example with HIV/AIDS (Weeks et al., 1996) and drug abuse (Mold and Berridge, 2008). Anecdotally, there is evidence of a greater interest in prevention and health promotion among cancer organizations and heart disease groups in recent years, reflected in their involvement in public health campaigns (for example, restrictions on smoking in public places). Similarly, mental health groups have been involved in campaigns to prevent mental illness, for example by addressing issues such as stress in the workplace. Baggott and Jones (2011) found that there was a higher than expected level of interest in public health issues among HCPOs (with around 60 per cent of groups stating that campaigning and lobbying on these issues was important). This may reflect broader policy agendas concerning the importance of helping people to maintain health and avoid illness.

Nonetheless, it is difficult to generalize about the relationship between government and the wider voluntary health sector given the absence of systematic studies. There are cases where groups have built up a strong positive relationship with policy-makers and have influenced public health policy. Examples include Cancer Research UK's campaign on the regulation of sunbeds. Other groups have antagonized government by campaigning for stronger policies (Action on Smoking and Health, the Alcohol Health Alliance, and Sustain, for example) but still exerted some influence over policy, as campaigns to regulate smoking and tobacco, prevent alcohol misuse and improve the quality of school food illustrate (Baggott, 2010a). However, these successful cases may not represent the true picture. As with HCPOs, the wider voluntary health sector appears to be diverse and unequal in the distribution of political, social and economic resources. For many of the smaller and less well-connected groups, establishing a strong relationship with government and other policy-making bodies and exerting influence over policy is a distant dream. Many prefer to focus instead on providing information, support and advice for their particular client group or membership.

Local voluntary health organizations

Our understanding of local relationships between voluntary health organizations and statutory health agencies and partnerships has also been hampered by a lack of studies. Most of the available evidence is drawn from studies of broader issues (such as community development or patient and public involvement) or specific policy issues or services (such as Sure Start or Health Action Zones). One exception is Wood's (2000) analysis of local patient organizations in Manchester. Wood's research explored local branches of national organizations. Moreover, he was primarily interested in internal structures, membership and the services provided, rather than their engagement with statutory agencies. Nonetheless, Wood's findings, that most local branches were modest in size, had limited financial resources and were volunteer-led and run by small committees, indicated the limited scale and capacity of these bodies. He found little in the way of collaboration between groups or of even low-level campaigning on health issues.

A more recent study (Willmott, 2012) explored the role of voluntary organizations in one local area and examined their relationships with local health bodies. Although a single case study, this nonetheless provided rich evidence about local groups and their relationship with decision-makers. Its findings confirmed some of the points made earlier, challenged some current assumptions and provide a basis for further studies. Willmott found that although not perceiving themselves as powerful, voluntary organizations in the health arena regarded themselves and were regarded by local agencies as legitimate participants in the local policy process. They had relevant expertise and knowledge. They were also able to speak on behalf of a group of patients (and mediate between agencies and patients). However, resource constraints on such groups were evident and represented a barrier to participation. Willmott also found that, in some policy areas, there was an element of selection at work: NHS bodies controlled which groups could be involved. Both selection and resource constraints meant that there was bias against less well-funded and smaller organizations and those that did not have good relationships with the NHS and local government. The incorporation of groups and public funding was used as a means of control. However, groups that provided specialized services could exert leverage as the NHS came to depend on them. Although being a service provider enhanced access to policy-makers and yielded opportunities to influence, service providers moderated their policy advocacy to preserve their status with policy-makers. Willmott found a limited degree of collaboration between groups, and some tensions (arising in part from competitive pressure between groups). However, the local voluntary service umbrella organization acted as a mediator between voluntary organizations and NHS bodies, and as a representative and advocate for the sector. Interestingly, Willmott's study revealed the potential for tensions between the parallel systems of voluntary sector engagement and public and patient involvement.

The study identified multiple opportunities for voluntary organizations to engage in local health policy processes and identified several issues that stimulated opportunities for engagement. These included developments in commissioning, the statutory duty on the NHS to involve patients and the public, as well as the current health policy agenda (the emergence of some issues on the policy agenda could create opportunities for organizations that focused on those issues). Voluntary organizations tended to press for incremental change and, like Wood, Willmott found no evidence of radical protest. However, she found that some groups were attempting to push boundaries, notably with regard to strengthening the focus on prevention issues and public health.

Although systematic studies are thin on the ground, one can find many examples of voluntary health organizations shaping local policies, influencing planning and delivering services (Box 6.2). It is clear from the scraps of evidence – often gleaned indirectly from wider studies of partnership arrangements, policies and programmes – that voluntary health organizations have encountered obstacles when seeking to influence local planning and service delivery. In one survey, less than half of local patient organizations were involved with health commissioning in their local area (Patient View, 2009). By the same token, local health decision-makers have faced difficulties when genuinely seeking to engage with the sector.

The problems facing the voluntary health sector reflect the broader issues encountered by the sector. A key problem is lack of capacity. This was identified by a major study of public health partnerships, which found that although the voluntary sector was increasingly important, there was a lack of capacity and this represented a major barrier to partnership working (Hunter et al., 2011). Others have found that voluntary health organizations could strengthen their position, for example by improving their ability to gather and share data and research relating to population health, to engage with policy-makers and to sell their services to commissioners, with appropriate support (ACEVO, 2010; Curry et al., 2011). Studies of Health Action Zones noted that engagement with NHS and other local agencies placed a considerable burden on the officers and representatives of voluntary health organizations (Unwin and Westland, 2000; Matka et al., 2002).

An improvement in the capacity of service planners and managers to engage with the voluntary sector needed was also needed, according to some. More specifically, a failure to engage voluntary health organizations fully in needs assessment and planning has been found (ACEVO, 2010; Curry et al., 2011; Harding and Kane, 2011).

Box 6.2	Voluntary organizations in public health

Voluntary organizations have been involved in a range of health and well-being initiatives and projects at local level. For example, local alliances to tackle smoking have included voluntary groups. Voluntary organizations have also been involved in programmes at local level to reduce teenage pregnancy, sexually transmitted disease and drug and alcohol misuse, and to promote healthy eating and exercise. Initiatives such as Healthy Living Centres, Sure Start, Healthy Communities and Health Action Zones have also included the voluntary sector. Voluntary organizations were included in Healthy Cities projects and in the Healthy Towns programme. They have also been involved in projects to improve the health of older people, children and ethnic groups, and in initiatives to reduce health inequalities.

The diversity of public health activities involving the voluntary sector is illustrated by the projects funded by the DH's Communities for Health programme. Of the 82 local areas that reported on how they spent their allocation, 45 explicitly mentioned working with voluntary organizations, community groups or social enterprises. Projects included promoting mental health, encouraging people to adopt healthy lifestyles, improving healthy eating, encouraging the take-up of sport, tackling obesity, smoking cessation, preventing alcohol problems and improving sexual health. Involvement varied from being consulted, being involved in planning groups and jointly running events to directly delivering services. Although many of these projects were evaluated, there is little publicly available evidence on how the voluntary sector impacted on the cost-effectiveness of the schemes.

A flavour of the kind of work that is being done, exemplifying best practice in the field, can be derived from beacon schemes and awards such as the GSK/King's Fund Impact Awards. Examples of projects involving the voluntary sector are given below:

Project 6 (Keighley, West Yorkshire). Based in an area of deprivation, a voluntary agency has worked with the local NHS and other agencies to reduce the harm caused by alcohol and drugs. It is an open access service that provides a range of services including advice, support, treatment, resettlement and aftercare. It includes an integrated family service and help for pregnant drug users, and provides services that are tailored to the needs of the South Asian community (see www.project6.org.uk).

Step Forward (Tower Hamlets, London). Based in an area of deprivation, this provides a person-centred holistic advice, counselling, personal development and family support service for young people covering issues such as housing, careers, education, emotional issues, difficulties at home and school, and mental health. It also provides a weekly sexual health clinic for people aged 11–25 years. Operating from a 'shop front' premises, it also undertakes outreach work in the community and in schools (see www.step-forward.web.org).

HealthWORKS (Newcastle, Tyneside). Based in two health resource centres, this organization seeks to enable people to take control over their own lives and adopt healthy lifestyles. It provides programmes to improve health and fitness, delivers information and advice, acts as a venue for other providers with similar aims, and works in partnership with statutory agencies and other programmes such as health trainers and Change4Life (see www.hwn.org.uk).

With regard to service provision, it appears that some voluntary health organizations are unable to compete for contracts effectively without considerable support. Curry et al. (2011) found that smaller organizations faced particular problems in this regard (see also Voluntary Action Westminster, 2010, for a local illustration). Larger organizations had more chance of success in winning contracts but sometimes lacked knowledge of the local community. In this context, the Association of Chief Executives of Voluntary Organizations (ACEVO, 2010) identified greater scope for voluntary sector provision, especially in public health services, where it believed the market was currently underdeveloped.

Some public health and related programmes have engaged the voluntary sector more effectively than others. For example, some Sure Start programmes and children's centres have been run by voluntary organizations. In others, the voluntary sector played a major role in providing services and was strongly represented on Sure Start management boards (Tunstill et al., 2002). However, there have been problems, particularly for smaller voluntary groups with a limited capacity for attending meetings and getting their voices heard (Myers et al., 2004). Indeed, some voluntary organizations felt excluded and squeezed out, particularly following the transfer of responsibility for children's centres to local authorities (Children, School and Families Committee, 2010). In addition, there have been pressures on voluntary organizations to conform to criteria set by local authorities (Hodgson, 2004). The experience of Healthy Living Centres provided further evidence of voluntary sector involvement (Hills et al., 2007), with some good examples of strong statutory–voluntary sector collaboration. But these tended to emerge where there was a history of close collaboration. Moreover, there were important variations, a focus on community development being stronger in some schemes than others.

Other problems include short-term funding and bureaucratic funding arrangements (see ACEVO, 2010; Voluntary Action Westminster, 2010). Issues of independence have also been raised. As voluntary health organizations are drawn into institutional structures and receive funding, they become constrained and have to conform to procedures often not suited to their own governance structures (Unwin and Westland, 2000). Another commonly identified problem is an unsystematic approach to engaging with the voluntary sector (see Barnes et al., 2007). This reflects broader issues concerning relationships between government institutions and the voluntary sector referred to earlier in this chapter in the context of central and local government. Previous studies of health service engagement have found that community involvement in practice tended to mean the involvement of 'known' individuals often from high-profile voluntary organizations (Jewkes and Murcott, 1998). Given the diversity of the voluntary health sector, there are dangers in relying on a few groups to represent the entire sector. This means that other groups may be under-represented or even misrepresented in engagement processes.

Nonetheless, as was pointed out earlier in this chapter, current health reforms hold several opportunities for the voluntary sector to shape public health policies and services in the future. Guidance has been provided for voluntary organizations to help them navigate and respond to these developments and maximize their input (Compact Voice, 2012; Regional Voices, 2012). In some parts of the country, systems of interaction have been established with the voluntary sector on health matters, encouraging collaboration within the sector and between public health decision-makers and voluntary organizations. For example, in Leicester-shire, a new voluntary and community strategy group was established coordinate and support the sector's input into an integrated commissioning framework (Kuznetsova, 2012).

Conclusion

Over the past three decades, policies and political factors have brought the voluntary sector more closely into the policy process and service provision. However, the sector has been prevented from fulfilling its potential as a partner for several reasons, including problems relating to capacity, funding regimes and engagement with government and public authorities. In particular, there has been a failure to deal adequately with the tensions between the voluntary organization's roles of advocate, representative and service provider. Moreover, inequalities within the sector need to be addressed. A further issue is the lack of consideration by authorities of the burden placed on voluntary organizations by their engagement in strategy and service provision. These problems have been compounded by the scepticism surrounding the 'Big Society' and the impact of other government policies on the ability of the voluntary sector to promote and support this agenda.

These broader issues have affected voluntary organizations focusing on health and well-being. Their contribution to health improvement and disease prevention is well documented. But it is also clear that this potential is not being fully realized. Voluntary organizations and other third sector bodies are legitimate partners in public health and well-being, and more must be done to strengthen their representative, advocacy and service provision roles, and to resolve potential conflicts of interest between them.

7 Partnerships with the private sector

Introduction

Increasingly, the private sector (businesses, commercial organizations and for-profit organizations) is seen as an important partner in public health and well-being. This chapter explores the role of the private sector in some depth. It begins by discussing the potential for involving business in partnerships to improve health and well-being. This is followed by a discussion of the drawbacks and problems of private sector involvement. The next section focuses on the role of the private sector in health partnerships at global level. This is followed by a review of recent national policies on the private sector and public health in the UK, including the Coalition government's Responsibility Deal. Finally, some examples of local partnership working with the private sector are discussed. The chapter also considers the role of social enterprises in health and well-being (see Box 7.1).

Business, health and well-being

An enemy rather than an ally?

Historically, business has often been depicted as the enemy of public health. This view is closely linked to the unhealthy living and working conditions of industrialization (Wohl, 1984). One can find many cases of blind and blatant self-interest from this period, such as the resistance of water companies to improvements in sanitation (Finer, 1952), and commercial opposition to quarantines because of their effect on trade (Longmate, 1966). To be fair, even in the heyday of laissez-faire capitalism, the private sector contributed to public health and well-being, through rising levels of economic prosperity and employment, improvements in conditions of work (pioneered by enlightened employers), civic works and philanthropy. In more recent times, it has been acknowledged that the private sector can contribute to health and well-being, both directly and in partnership with other stakeholders (Hancock, 1998; Simon and Fielding, 2006). In addition to its role in promoting health through rising economic standards and employment, there are two main contributions that the private sector can make: to act as responsible producers and employers, regulating their own behaviour, and to supply specific prevention services and products.

Corporate social responsibility and self-regulation

In the past, the standard response to allegations that business was damaging public health was denial, coupled with resistance to state regulation. This road was taken by the asbestos and tobacco industries, for example, in their reaction to evidence that serious diseases were linked to their products. While business still harbours a largely negative view of state regulation, the approach today is not to ignore or reject such issues, but rather to acknowledge and respond to them. This approach has been endorsed by key reports on public health in recent years. Wanless (2007) pointed out that the private sector had a duty to provide clear, consistent and relevant communication on issues of safety, content and the health impact of its products. Wanless also believed that businesses should promote health by offering healthy choices to consumers, while the Nuffield Commission on Bioethics (2007) concluded that this was an ethical duty.

An acknowledgement that business can help to improve health and well-being is linked to the broader notion of corporate social responsibility (CSR). CSR involves an acceptance that businesses have responsibilities to staff, customers, the wider public and government that go beyond the narrow generation of profits for shareholders (Carroll, 1999; Manokha, 2004; Horrigan, 2010). Many corporations have now adopted CSR, including companies in industries such as alcohol, food and tobacco. CSR is not without its critics – including those argue that the profit motive is the only true moral imperative of business (Friedman, 1970), as well as sceptics who see it as a little more than a public relations exercise (see below). Although CSR is a modern term, businesses have long engaged in similar activities to maintain and enhance their public reputation.

A key aspect of corporate responsibility is self-regulation, where businesses regulate their own behaviour to maintain standards of practice. This too has a long history, and in many countries, including the UK, there is a tradition of self-regulation, especially in fields such as the professions, skilled trades and business (Baggott, 1989; Better Regulation Task Force, 1999). Self-regulatory systems vary according to their autonomy from the state, by the legal force of their rules and in their ability to control entry to a particular market (Ogus, 1997). It is not uncommon for self-regulation to be underpinned by legislation and for the state to actively engage in establishing, endorsing and reforming self-regulatory systems (Moran, 2003). Indeed, many regulatory systems today are more accurately described as 'co-regulation' (Grabosky and Braithwaite, 1986) as they involve aspects of both state and self-regulation.

One of the main putative advantages of self-regulation over direct state regulation is that it harnesses the knowledge and expertise of those being regulated. Other advantages include: that self-regulation is based on consensus and is likely to improve compliance; that the spirit as well as the letter of the law is likely to be upheld; and that it is less costly to government and may possibly place a lesser burden on the regulated as well. Furthermore, it is believed that self-regulation is more flexible than direct regulation and more responsive to new and changing conditions.

As will become clear later, public health policy-makers have favoured a particular instrument of self-regulation, the voluntary agreement (Baggott, 1986; Storey et al., 1999). Voluntary agreements between government and industry aim to persuade the latter to undertake activities in pursuit of social goals. They are often used instead of direct intervention but in some cases are underpinned by statute (for example, health and safety codes of practice). It is difficult to generalize about them, as they are often tailored to a specific context. However, they appear to be most effective when they set clear targets, are subject to robust monitoring, involve third parties (that is, not just the industry and government but public or representatives of non-government organizations [NGOs]), include information-oriented benefits (such as technical forums where all parties can learn from experience), involve sanctions for non-compliance, and pose a credible threat of legislation or direct state action should voluntary approaches fail.

Private sector involvement in public health programmes

There are several possible advantages arising from private sector involvement in health improvement and disease prevention programmes (Hancock, 1998; Simon and Fielding, 2006, Sturchio and Goel, 2012). Companies may be involved in the manufacture of drugs or other products that prevent illness or promote health (such as vaccines or screening equipment). Also, as Wanless (2007) noted, private sector suppliers can strengthen the capacity of the public health system to support healthier behaviours, for example, in the case of obesity, private sport and leisure facilities and weight loss services. The private sector can bring resources, financial, human or technical, which may help to develop more effective prevention programmes. For example, a business may donate funds to bodies or campaigns to reduce a particular health problem, or may allow its staff to be seconded to specific campaigns (for example, alcohol company marketing experts contributing to sensible drinking campaigns). The involvement of the private sector may build a consensus through a 'round-table' approach with government and other policy actors and experts. By involving business in this way, it is possible that other stake-holders might reach a better understanding of its position, while business may obtain greater insights into the concerns of health professionals and campaigners, ultimately leading to more effective and better implemented policies. As employers, businesses may further contribute to health improvement by establishing healthy lifestyle programmes for their workers.

Disadvantages of working with the private sector

Power, CSR and self-regulation

Many of the disadvantages of private sector involvement are rooted in fears about its motives and power. Industries such as food, alcohol and tobacco have exerted much influence over government (Taylor, 1984; Baggott, 1990; Lang and Heasman, 2004; Lang et al., 2009; Miller and Harkins, 2010; Cairney et al., 2012; Hawkins et al., 2012). Industry often has a conflict of interest on health matters: it may genuinely wish to reduce health problems while at the same time seeking to profit from products that cause these problems (Gilmore and Fooks, 2012). There are suspicions that businesses seek to influence partnerships only to further their commercial ends. Notably, the alcohol and food industries have used partnership forums to oppose state regulation. Such partnerships tend to focus on the 'consensual' end of the policy spectrum, such as health education, which tends to be ineffective when used in isolation, rather than more controversial and potent policy instruments, such as controls on price and availability (Babor et al., 2003). A related issue is that partnership working arrangements give industry a foot in the door and enable it to exert power over other participants, especially the voluntary sector (Sklair and Miller, 2010). Some see a corrupting tendency in big business as part of a deliberate strategy to undermine evidence-based policies and independent science, and capture government and partnership bodies (McGarrity and Wagner, 2008; Miller and Harkins, 2010). Indeed, some take the view that the power of business is such that it should be isolated from policy formation (WHO Regional Office for Europe, 2006b), and that rather than working with business, the priority should be to advocate policies to challenge corporate power and modify its practices that damage health (Freudenberg, 2012; Hastings, 2012).

Critics see CSR as an important public relations tool (Bakan, 2005; Sklair and Miller, 2010). For them, corporations remain accountable primarily to shareholders, distorting their decision-making and leading them to operate against the wider public interest. Although businesses are worried about criticism, which can affect consumer and shareholder confidence, profits will always dominate their calculations because of the intrinsic nature of the corporation and its primary duty to shareholders. CSR offers a way of managing public perceptions. It is, however, more than a public relations tool. It strengthens the legitimacy of business groups outside its primary sphere of influence (economic, trade and fiscal policies). By taking an explicit position on health and welfare issues, and by adopting a 'socially responsible' position, businesses can secure access to policy networks that determine policies affecting their markets (Miller and Harkins, 2010; Fooks, 2011; Gilmore and Fooks, 2012).

There is also some cynicism about businesses' charitable activities. In many cases, charitable foundations are genuinely philanthropic. However, businesses often set up trusts that address problems closely associated with its products. An example might be an alcohol company funding alcohol education programmes. Although on the surface this may appear philanthropic, such funds could be seen as 'blood money', with businesses continuing to profit from illness while making a relatively small contribution to the alleviation of problems they have caused. There are also concerns that companies can attach strings, ensuring that recipients of their largesse do not undermine their profitable activities, by for example campaigning for legislation restricting the marketing of their products.

Furthermore, there is much scepticism about self-regulation in public health (LGA et al., 2004; House of Lords Select Committee on Science and Technology,

2011). Critics highlight the disadvantage associated with self-regulatory systems in general: that self-regulation tends to be complacent and underenforced; that it lacks legitimacy and attracts suspicion that self-regulatory bodies are concerned primarily with protecting commercial interests; that there are few effective sanctions and limited powers for self-regulatory bodies to achieve compliance; that self-regulatory bodies are unable to influence non-members (unless there is compulsory membership or licensing system); that they often involve confusion of functions and conflicts of interest (such as between the regulatory versus the representational roles of trade bodies); that self-regulation is not as publicly accountable as state regulation; and that it can be costly, especially where there is a co-regulation element.

Public health services

While immunizations and other preventive drugs produced by the private sector have saved many lives, it is acknowledged that the drugs industry's main aim is profit. Many drug scandals – such as Thalidomide and Opren – have had severe public health consequences. There are also dangers of overmedication and the adoption of inappropriate pharmaceutical treatment in place of alternative therapies or actions to address the social and environmental causes of illness. An example might be the use of obesity drugs or surgery in favour of action to tackle to the obesogenic food environment. The same arguments apply to screening, which can be cost-effective but is not always so (see, for example, the controversy surrounding breast cancer screening; *Lancet*, 2012). Private companies make much money out of screening and health checks, both from the provision of equipment and by providing services to the NHS and private individuals. But there is mounting concern that many of these services may be unnecessary and therefore harmful. Particular disquiet surrounds the private 'health MOT' industry (see National Screening Committee, 2010).

Pragmatism

Others, while aware of the difficulties of getting the private sector to conform to public health principles and policy, are more pragmatic. One approach is to get private corporations to agree to specific principles of public health policy and standards of behaviour (Hancock, 1998). Where business falls short of the mark, additional state regulation may be introduced, and this threat may itself produce compliance (Nuffield Council on Bioethics, 2007). Furthermore, it may be possible to design partnership working arrangements to minimize problems, such as conflicts of interest (for example, business influence over public health campaigns and partnership bodies might be inhibited by the use of 'blind trusts', where business funds the activity but does not have say in decisions about policy or strategy).

Other recommendations concern self-regulation. There could be a greater emphasis on co-regulation. One suggestion is that there could be more external independent evaluation of self-regulation against clear objectives (House of Lords Select Committee on Science and Technology, 2011). This reflects the recommendations of the National Consumer Council (NCC, 2005) that self-regulatory systems generally should conform to the following principles: clear objectives, wide consultation about design and operation, a dedicated body to manage self-regulation (rather than a trade or professional association), a well-publicized complaints procedure, monitoring of compliance, adequate resourcing, effective sanctions, performance indicators and regular reviews to ensure the system is working. The National Consumer Council also emphasized the importance of independent members (who should be in a majority and ideally an independent chair) and that a self-regulatory system should be publicized so that the public were aware of its existence.

Another approach is to use business organization models to achieve public health objectives but, rather than operate on a purely 'for-profit' basis, establish them as social enterprises (Box 7.1).

Box 7.1 Social enterprises

According to the Department of Trade and Industry (2002, p. 13) 'a social enterprise is a business with primarily social objectives, whose surpluses are principally reinvested for that purpose in the business or in the community, rather than being driven by the need to maximize profits for shareholders and owners.' However, there is no widely accepted definition, which makes it difficult to map and study this sector (Lyon and Sepulveda, 2009). Indeed, the boundaries between what one might regard as a social enterprise and other organizations in the voluntary and private sectors is blurred (Marks and Hunter, 2007). Although the term is relatively new, social enterprises have existed in various forms for many years. For example, mutual building societies, provident insurance societies and cooperatives could all be considered as forms of social enterprise. More recently, social enterprise has been seen by political thinkers and governments as an important middle course between the state and the market. The New Labour governments of Blair and Brown backed social enterprise, as has the Coalition government of David Cameron. Indeed, the idea was attractive to those advocating the 'Big Society' (Blond, 2010; Norman, 2010).

In 2001, the New Labour government established a social enterprise unit within government. A strategy was launched in 2002 (entitled Strategy for Success), and a social enterprise action plan in 2006. Social enterprises were seen as a key part of the wider 'third sector' (see Chapter 6) that was particularly well placed to compete for public sector contracts. They were praised for their ability to respond flexibly to needs and innovate, and seen as enabling staff to have greater autonomy and be empowered to deliver a better service. The health and social care arena was identified as an area where social enterprises might flourish (Lewis et al., 2006; Addicott, 2011). The NHS was encouraged to transfer service provision to social enterprises, with a particular push to create employee-owned enterprises (Ham and Ellins, 2010). This emphasis continued under the Coalition government, which planned to open NHS services to greater competition from the independent sector (Cm 7985, 2010; Cm 8145, 2011).

Recent governments have encouraged social enterprise in the field of public health (Cm 6374, 2004; Cm 6737, 2006; ACEVO, 2010; Taylor et al., 2011). Social enterprises are currently involved in many areas of service delivery including the primary care services, healthy living centres, holistic health and well-being strategies, alcohol and substance misuse services, support for people with learning disabilities and long-term conditions, and health promotion programmes, and the provision of a range of health and social care services to groups such as vulnerable adults and homeless people. Social enterprises have also been involved in community engagement and patient and public involvement (see Chapter 5).

There have been concerns about social enterprises, both generally (Bull, 2008; Pattie and Johnston, 2011) and specifically in relation to health and care services (Marks and Hunter, 2007; Addicott, 2011; Taylor et al., 2011). There are fears that they are a vehicle for reducing the role of the state, privatization and cost-cutting. Another concern is that the transfer of work to social enterprise could undermine the terms and conditions of employees (although some protection has been promised). There are also concerns – reflecting similar issues across the voluntary sector – that social enterprises are ill equipped because of their size and scale to compete effectively for contracts. There are issues of risk and viability too. What happens to services if the social enterprise fails? Furthermore, pluralism in supply could lead to a greater fragmentation of services and a poorly coordinated service for the user.

Public–private partnerships at global level

During the late 1990s, the World Health Organization (WHO) highlighted the potential for involving the private sector as a partner in global health alliances (WHO, 1999). Private sector organizations were invited to participate in WHO conferences on health promotion, which made clear statements of intent that reflected the private sector's contribution. The 4th International Conference on Health Promotion in Jakarta (1997), for example, called for cooperation between all sectors, including the private sector, on health matters, and set out how private companies could contribute to health, for example by protecting the environment, restricting production and trade in harmful products, discouraging unhealthy marketing, and protecting workers. Subsequently, the Bangkok Conference in 2005 reiterated this, making it clear that the private sector was a legitimate partner in health promotion and should be held to account for its actions and their health consequences. Meanwhile, partnership with the private sector on health matters was being encouraged in international development policies. Between 1990 and 2010, annual development assistance for health more than quadrupled (from almost £6 billion to nearly £27 billion), much of this increase coming through public–private partnerships (Sturchio and Goel, 2012).

Public–private partnerships expanded in the context of a global pro-business ideology (Buse and Walt, 2000; Reich, 2000). This is likely to continue, given ongoing pressures to involve business in global health and development. Definitions and typologies of these arrangements were devised (Reich, 2000; Widdus, 2001; Nishtar, 2004). It was acknowledged that public–private partnerships varied considerably (Nishtar, 2004). Some were led by public organizations, others by the private sector. Some included NGOs. Their specific aims and objectives varied. Moreover, they could be found in different contexts, including product development (such as new drugs), improving access to care and treatment, health services reform, coordination of strategies, education and public advocacy, regulation and quality assurance (Widdus, 2001; Nishtar, 2004).

Specific examples of private involvement include global strategies on non-communicable diseases, including obesity and diet-related diseases, alcohol-related problems and environmental health (see Chapter 2), which have involved private corporations in their formulation and implementation. The private sector is also involved in arrangements for delivering prevention services, care and treatment, primarily to developing countries (see Brugha and Walt, 2001). For example, the Global Alliance for Vaccines and Immunisation (GAVI) has provided access to vaccines and drug treatments, as well as investing in health systems. GAVI includes UN agencies (the World Bank, WHO and UNICEF) governments, NGOs and drug companies. The Global Fund to Fight AIDS, Tuberculosis and Malaria targets these major infectious diseases, provides vaccines and drug treatments, and funds training. This programme also involves drug companies and NGOs, as well as international agencies and individual countries.

Given the diverse and often controversial nature of such partnerships, it is difficult to arrive at a balanced conclusion about them. However, it is possible to draw some conclusions. On the one hand, some partnerships promise significant potential benefits. For example, as noted elsewhere in this chapter, involving the private sector in health promotion can have significant advantages, bringing additional resources and expertise to bear on health problems (Hancock, 1998; Sturchio and Goel, 2012). In addition, it is possible that companies may become more socially responsible through their involvement in health issues, and may acknowledge health factors within their commercial practices (Kickbusch and Payne, 2004). There is also evidence that some partnerships have borne fruit (McKinsey and Co, 2002; Caines, 2004), raising the profile of particular diseases, accelerating efforts to prevent and treat illness, mobilizing resources and in some cases promoting innovation. Partnerships such as the GAVI Alliance and the Global Fund, although not without their shortcomings (see below), have increased access to life-saving vaccines and others drugs for millions of people (McCarthy, 2007; Arie, 2011).

Nonetheless, critics have identified a range of problems. Partnerships have been criticized for exhibiting weaknesses in governance, poor management systems, inefficiency, waste (and in some cases, where funding has been involved, fraud and corruption), lack of coordination and overlap with other initiatives, including other partnerships (Caines, 2004; Buse and Harmer, 2007). For example, both GAVI and the Global Fund have attracted criticism for weaknesses in governance and inefficiencies (McCarthy, 2007; Arie, 2011). There has also been concern that partnerships lack transparency and democratic accountability (Buse and Walt, 2000; Pinet, 2003; Nishtar, 2004). Another criticism is that partnerships are rarely evaluated, and even when they are, this is often short term, unsystematic and superficial, focusing more on the benefits than on the costs of partnership (Caines, 2004; Nishtar, 2004).

The power and influence of commercial organizations is a further issue. Global businesses have the power and political weight to lobby strongly at international level, blocking or diluting strategies and initiatives that threaten their profitability. They can also influence NGOs, setting up their own 'front organizations' (BINGOs – business interest NGOs – in contrast to PINGOs – public interest NGOs; see Conflicts of Interest Coalition, 2011). It is argued that corporations often have a conflict of interest when participating in partnerships. They have an incentive to engage in activities that limit or reduce public benefit in order to protect profits and sales (Buse and Walt, 2000; Nishtar, 2004; Fooks, 2011). For example, the GAVI scheme has been criticized for not doing enough to reduce the prices of essential drugs (Arie, 2011; *Private Eye*, 2011). Some industries are recognized as beyond the pale – notably tobacco – because their interests are seen as diametrically opposed to health. However, drugs companies, food and alcohol corporations and others that can contribute to better health and reduce the harm caused by their products are regarded by some as legitimate partners. Others, however, argue that their role should be strictly confined to the practical implementation of policy and should not be allowed to influence strategies (see below). An even more fundamental criticism is that public–private partnerships represent a shift away from public values towards commercial values, markets and privatization. There are fears that this corrupts public values and enables governments and international agencies to shift responsibility on to others (Buse and Waxman, 2001; Nishtar, 2004).

A range of other issues have also been raised (Buse and Walt, 2000; Brugha and Walt, 2001; Buse and Waxman, 2001; Caines, 2004; Nishtar, 2004), including the short-term nature of some partnerships and their lack of sustainability, the focus on specific diseases rather than holistic issues of public health and well-being and the provision of comprehensive healthcare, and, in the case of international health aid, the imposition of Western 'solutions' on to developing countries, undermining their autonomy and responsibility.

In order to yield the benefits of partnership, it is important that these issues are fully addressed (Buse and Harmer, 2007). Critics have pressed for key principles and norms for public–private partnerships, addressing issues such as governance, conflicts of interest, accountability, openness and transparency (Pinet, 2003; Nishtar, 2004). They have argued in favour of much stronger frameworks within which partnerships can develop and operate (Buse and Walt, 2000). The UN introduced a Global Compact in 2007, setting out 10 principles for business, based on core values of human rights, labour standards, environment and anti-corruption (UN, 2007). Principles include 'businesses should support and respect the protection of internationally proclaimed human rights', 'businesses should support a precautionary approach to environmental challenges' and 'businesses should work against corruption in all its forms, including extortion and bribery'. The WHO, which has endorsed these principles, has its own guidelines on interaction with commercial enterprises (WHO, 2000b). Although these bar the most obvious abuses (such as the donation of cash from a company with direct commercial interests, the use of the WHO's logo in advertising, and secondments from companies whose activities clearly conflict with the WHO's mandate), processes of enforcement are unclear. Aside from complaints about specific abuses, there is no system for monitoring or regulating compliance. Nor is there a clear and effective mechanism for punishing transgressors.

There is little to stop unethical businesses from operating in partnerships in ways damaging to health. Reforming partnerships is one way forward, but some doubt that the private sector can act ethically and that its participation in health partnerships is dangerous. Certainly, there is evidence that private enterprise, often in league with neoliberal governments, has been able to lobby successfully for policies that benefit them (Lee and Collin, 2005; *Lancet*, 2011; Stuckler et al., 2011), and evidence of serious conflicts of interest in relationships between the private sector and international agencies (Cohen and Carter, 2010; Corporate Accountability International, 2011; *Private Eye*, 2011). Arguments can be made that, in some areas of policy at least, partnerships are inappropriate. In others, the private sector's role may need to be restricted. In this regard, the Conflicts of Interest Coalition (2011) has proposed a framework to be used as a code of conduct for industry, which states that the policy development stage should be free of industry involvement. However, it is acknowledged that companies may be briefed on policy (although not allowed to lobby) and that they can have a role in policy implementation.

UK policies on public health and the private sector

Business involvement in public health policies is not entirely a modern phenomenon. Suppliers of health products and services have long worked in partnership with national governments. For example, the drugs industry has enjoyed a close relationship with the UK government on issues such as drug pricing, research and development, and the availability of drugs, particularly in emergencies. Moreover, government has held discussions with business (as well as public sector employers and trade unions) on workplace health issues such as the prevention of accidents and, more recently, on the promotion of mental and physical health. Industries whose products have been linked to ill health, such as food, tobacco and alcohol, have also worked with government for many years. In the 1970s, the government and the tobacco industry established voluntary agreements covering matters such as product modification and marketing (Taylor, 1984). These were heavily criticized by anti-smoking campaigners, who pressed for legislation to ban tobacco advertising and to have tobacco regulated as a dangerous substance. In recent years, this voluntary approach has been replaced with a stronger emphasis on legislative intervention, with bans on tobacco advertising and sponsorship and prohibitions on smoking in public places, alongside tougher fiscal policies, hard-hitting health education campaigns and smoking cessation services (Cairney et al., 2012).

The drinks industry has also engaged extensively with government to deter stronger policies to limit alcohol consumption (Baggott, 1990). The industry has long feared the imposition of price controls, tax increases and restrictions on the availability and marketing of its products. It has negotiated codes of practice governing advertising and marketing since the 1970s. In 1996, it introduced its own self-regulatory system for the promotion of alcoholic drinks in response to the growing disquiet about 'alcopops', fruit-flavoured ready-to-drink alcohol products that appealed to younger people. This code was introduced and managed by the industry's 'social responsibility' body, the Portman Group, established in

1989 to bring together existing social responsibility initiatives and pre-empt direct government regulation (Baggott, 2006).

The food industry has interacted with government on concerns about the nutritional content of food, particularly high fat, salt and sugar levels, and on other issues such as food safety, and genetically modified and novel foods. In the 1980s and 1990s, the industry exerted much influence, leading government to suppress key scientific advisory reports that proposed targets for healthier food and nutrition. The bodies that made uncomfortable recommendations for industry were then abolished or reconstituted. The government agreed that a voluntary approach was most appropriate, and this took the form of voluntary labelling schemes and minor restrictions on advertising (Mills, 1992). However, as levels of obesity began to grow, it became more difficult for the industry to close down debate and block policies that threatened its economic interests.

New Labour and the private sector

Although New Labour's initial health policies largely ignored the role of the private sector in the provision of care and treatment services, and was hostile to some industries (notably tobacco, for which it adopted much stronger anti-smoking policies than its predecessor), this position shifted dramatically within a few years of taking office. The NHS Plan of 2000 (Cm 4818, 2000), and a subsequent agreement between the Department of Health (DH) and the independent sector, heralded a new era in which private providers would be offered greater opportunities to work in partnership with the NHS and provide health and social care services funded by the taxpayer. This shift was reflected in public health policies too. Although *Saving Lives*, Labour's first public health White Paper, barely mentioned the private sector (Cm 4386, 1999), subsequent policy documents identified the private sector as a key partner in delivering public health objectives. *Choosing Health* (Cm 6374, 2004) outlined how the private sector could shape opportunities for physical activity and healthy eating, for example highlighting the role of catering companies in influencing food choices. It urged greater corporate responsibility, particularly by food and alcoholic drink companies in the marketing of their products. In addition, occupational health and support for employees in both private and public sector organizations was encouraged.

In relation to alcohol, there was astonishment that *Choosing Health* proposed delegating key responsibilities to the Portman Group (Baggott, 2006). Some saw this body as merely a front for the drinks industry (Edwards et al., 2004), or as lobbyist (Harkins, 2010), which it strenuously denied (Coussins, 2004). There was also scepticism about the Portman Group's role in relation to self-regulation and alcohol health education (Mayor, 2004; Baggott, 2006). Following the publication of its alcohol strategy (Prime Minister's Strategy Unit, 2004), the government created a new body, the Drinkaware Trust, governed jointly by the drinks industry and independent members. This administered existing funds for educational and community projects to reduce alcohol misuse that had formerly fallen under the auspices of the Portman Group, along with additional funds from the industry and other sources (such as the Big Lottery). In addition, government and the industry agreed a set of national standards on social responsibility, covering issues such as sensible drinking, underage drinking and marketing. A voluntary industry code on alcohol labelling was also introduced. Amid concerns about binge drinking, the impact of extending licensing hours (introduced by New Labour in the Licensing Act 2003) and adverse findings from evaluations of the national social responsibility standards and the labelling code (Baggott, 2010b), the government responded with a more robust approach. This included restrictions on the new licensing laws, increasing penalties for breaches of the law, and higher taxes on alcohol (HM Government, 2007b). Nonetheless, the influence of the industry over policy remained strong (BMA, 2009; Health Committee, 2010).

There was a similar story in the area of food, nutrition and obesity. Although New Labour established a new system of food safety and nutrition standards under the Food Standards Agency (FSA), it shied away from policy instruments such as tax and legislative restrictions that were opposed by industry. Instead, health promotion education campaigns were pursued, notably Change4Life (C4L), which was primarily aimed at getting individuals and families to take responsibility for their own health (see Chapter 5). Businesses did contribute to C4L (by, for example, giving discounts on healthier food products), but the scheme was consistent with commercial interests, as it enhanced businesses' corporate images, helped them market their products and pre-empted direct state interventions. Notably, a similar scheme was proposed by the food and advertising industry prior to the policy initiative being announced (Miller and Harkins, 2010).

However, the government was forced to strengthen regulation in a number of areas. School meal regulations were tightened in response to a powerful media campaign led by the celebrity chef Jamie Oliver. Rules on broadcasting advertising of food aimed at children were strengthened, again due to strong pressure from health campaigners. But the main emphasis of policy remained upon voluntary efforts and self-regulation. This was evident from the close working relationship between the FSA and the industry, and the use of voluntary targets to reduce levels of fat, salt and energy (including sugars) in food and drink. The government also adopted a voluntary approach to labelling, allowing companies to adopt schemes other than the 'traffic light' labelling system preferred by public health campaigners, although to be fair the government's hands were tied to a large extent here by European Union rules on food labelling. There were some positive outcomes, as levels of these ingredients did decline. Salt consumption fell substantially – by around 15 per cent between 2000 and 2010 – although this was not sufficient to meet the government's maximum recommended levels. Saturated fat and sugar consumption levels fell marginally, and also remained above maximum recommended levels.

Further cooperation between the government and the private sector was proposed by the Darzi Review (Cm 7432, 2008), which called for the establishment of a Coalition for Better Health, to involve industry and voluntary organizations in health promotion and the prevention of health problems. The initial focus was on obesity, but other areas included alcohol, health and work, and physical activity. Working groups were established to take forward initiatives identified by business and voluntary sector stakeholders. However, little in the way of new policy developments occurred as a result.

The Coalition government and the Responsibility Deal

The Coalition built on the previous government's policy by introducing a Responsibility Deal (RD), a set of agreements with industry and other stakeholders to address public health problems. This owed much to Conservative Party initiatives in opposition. A working party on CSR recommended the use of responsibility deals (Conservative Party, 2008) and identified a key role for government as a 'facilitator' of such arrangements, convening stakeholders, identifying common interests, negotiating cooperative and mutually beneficial strategies, and developing and in some cases overseeing institutions that managed and implemented these strategies. Andrew Lansley, then Shadow Health Secretary and later Secretary of State for Health under the Coalition, was keen to establish a framework of voluntary agreements between government and business on public health issues. He established a Public Health Commission, chaired by the chairman of Unilever, a major food and drinks producer. Its members included representatives of the food and drinks industry, alcohol producers, retailers, advertising, the fitness industry, consumer bodies and health charities, as well as nutritional, medical and other scientific experts. The Commission's report focused on several key issues – health in the workplace, alcohol misuse, nutrition and exercise – and made recommendations on how these problems could be tackled (Public Health Commission, 2009). The tone of the report reflected a preference for self-regulation by business, voluntary approaches to improving health, partnership with business and employers, and social marketing to promote individual behaviour change. A later Conservative Party (2010b) document further endorsed the principle that business, alongside the public and voluntary sectors, should be a joint owner of long-term public health strategy, and reiterated an intention to introduce an RD.

The emphasis on CSR chimed with the Coalition's support for ways of 'nudging' individuals into making positive health choices rather than imposing measures to restrict their liberty. This policy reflected New Labour's 'choosing health' approach and its C4L social marketing campaign (see Chapter 5). Drawing on ideas from a number of academics, 'nudging' is about changing the environment in which personal choices are made (Thaler and Sunstein, 2009). However, the evidence that it can change behaviour in the absence of regulatory measures is weak (Bonell, A. et al., 2011; Loewenstein et al., 2012).

These various factors led to the formulation of an RD with business and other organizations (from the voluntary and public sectors). The RD focused on alcohol, food, physical activity, and health at work and was developed by specific networks whose membership included businesses and trade associations, as well as voluntary health organizations, consumer groups, public sector representatives and scientific experts. A fifth, cross-cutting, network, on behaviour change, was also established. In addition, a plenary group was established, chaired by the Secretary of State for Health, to oversee the RD as a whole. Under the terms of the RD, organizations (from the voluntary sector as well as business) were asked to sign up to core commitments, collective and individual pledges, and supporting pledges (DH, 2011d). The five core commitments were that an organization would: recognize that it has a vital role in improving health; encourage and enable people to adopt a healthier diet; foster a culture of responsible drinking that will help people to drink within guidelines; encourage and assist people to become more physically active; and actively support its workforce to lead healthier lives. Collective and individual pledges set out actions that organizations would be expected to deliver against the core commitments. Collective pledges were designed by the networks, and each organization was expected to sign up to at least one collective pledge. In addition, individual pledges could be made by organizations (or subgroups of organizations), subject to approval by the chairs of each network and the DH. Collective pledges included: providing calorie information on food and non-alcoholic drinks in out-of-home settings, ensuring that the majority (80 per cent) of alcohol products had clear labelling of units, NHS guidelines and health warnings about drinking in pregnancy; contributing to the communication and promotion of the Chief Medical Officer's revised physical activity guidelines; and ensuring healthier staff restaurants. These and other pledges are examined in more detail below in relation to the specific sectors covered by the RD.

Five 'supporting pledges' were formulated to underpin the collective and individual pledges. These were: to support the RD and encourage other organizations to sign up; to acknowledge that the RD's strength comes from organizations of different types across varying sectors working together to improve health; to contribute to the monitoring and evaluation of progress against the pledges; when offering information about healthier choices, to ensure that this was consistent with government public health advice; and to broaden and deepen the impact of the RD by working to develop further pledges in support of the five core commitments.

Criticism of the RD

Meanwhile, a groundswell of opposition began to build. There was criticism of the principles behind the policy. For seasoned public health campaigners, and many scientific experts and NGOs, the idea of giving powerful business corporations a strong position within public health policy was incredibly dangerous. Although other stakeholders were included in the RD networks, they were outnumbered by people drawn from business. Furthermore, the networks' agendas were dominated by industry, and some non-business participants were concerned that they were simply legitimizing policy. As will become clear further on in this chapter, some non-industry groups, concerned particularly about the weaknesses of the RD in relation to food and alcoholic drink, refused to sign up.

There was disquiet about the vague nature of some of the commitments and pledges. The approach taken was not systematic, as some pledges set timescales for achievement and others did not. Few pledges set a clear target to be achieved (setting out what had to be achieved by when). Indeed, only three of the original 19 collective pledges set a clear deadline for achieving a goal. There was particular concern that many pledges were minimal, or of marginal importance, and provided a useful way for business to appear responsible without having to concede much ground (Boseley et al., 2011). Furthermore, although businesses (and other partners) were required to sign up to core commitments and supporting pledges, they did not have to endorse all the collective pledges, nor were they required to make individual pledges above and beyond collective pledges. This meant that a business could be seen in a positive light by becoming a partner in the RD but might actually sign up to only a single collective pledge. Furthermore, it was theoretically possible for a business in one of the more controversial sectors covered by the RD (that is, food and alcohol) to sign up to pledges in the less controversial areas (that is, health at work and physical activity). They could then represent themselves as a socially responsible partner, without having to address the primary public health issues arising from their corporate activities.

In addition, the RD did not mention sanctions should an organization breach its promises. For example, there was no process for 'de-registering' those who failed to meet commitments and pledges. Although the DH made it clear that progress would be monitored and that organizations must comply with an evaluation process, there were doubts about how robust this would be. The initial approach was to urge participants to report progress on pledges on an annual basis to the DH. This rather vague and weak approach fostered even more disquiet. The DH later agreed to an independent evaluation (funded through its Policy Research Programme). Another problem was that the RD was formulated in the absence of clear policy framework. Although the government published its White Paper on public health in November 2011, a few months before the launch of the RD, important strategies on obesity and alcohol were still being formulated. Such poor timing heightened the suspicion of health campaigners that the voluntary approach embedded in the RD was actually the main instrument of policy. Although the government denied this, and made it clear that key strategies would follow, this was not well communicated, which fuelled criticism.

The Health Secretary defended his approach (Lansley, 2011), stating that business had a legitimate role to play in health improvement. He denied that business had undue influence. He also stated that the RD was a first step in bringing businesses and other organizations on board and that it would evolve and develop. First, he expected that more businesses (and other organizations) would sign up. Second, he envisaged that, in future, new commitments and pledges would be added, strengthening the impact of the RD on public health. Moreover, he added that the RD was one strand of the government's policy on public health and would be complemented by other policies and interventions. Lansley was backed by the Chief Medical Officer, Sally Davies (White, 2011), who endorsed the RD and acknowledged that businesses had important expertise and skills, in marketing and sales for example, that could be deployed in preventing illness and promoting health. In 2011, further endorsement was forthcoming when the RD achieved a prestigious Civil Service Award for its efforts in promoting collaboration. The DH was able to point out that the RD had achieved significant agreement on a range of issues including alcohol labelling and the presentation of calorific content on food and drink. A total of 170 organizations (private, public and voluntary sector) initially endorsed the RD. By mid-2012, around 400 organizations had signed up, which government claimed was a major indication of success. The number of collective pledges also increased – to 26 by January 2013.

Alcohol

In addition to the criticism of the government's overall approach, there was much concern about specific aspects of the RD and its networks. The commitments and pledges on alcohol misuse proved the most controversial. Six organizations (Alcohol Concern, the British Association for the Study of the Liver, the British Medical Association, the British Liver Trust, the Institute of Alcohol Studies and the Royal College of Physicians) refused to endorse the alcohol deal. These groups were critical of the weakness of the pledges, some of which were seen as recycled versions of existing commitments. They also argued that there was an absence of policy on issues such as the pricing, regulation and availability of alcohol. Although the government was committed to an alcohol strategy in the light of party manifesto commitments and Coalition pledges on alcohol misuse, the RD was seen as putting the cart before the horse, and setting a dangerous course for future policy. In short, critics felt that the industry exerted far too much influence over policy. In addition to the six organizations that refused to endorse the RD, others (including the Faculty of Public Health and Cancer Research UK) made clear their reservations but nonetheless signed up.

The key pledges related to alcohol were on labelling (already mentioned above), the provision of consistent information through bars and other retailers in the alcohol trade about the unit content of drinks and how communication about drinking guidelines and harms could be improved, calorie labelling, preventing underage sales (through existing schemes such as Challenge 21 and Challenge 25), support for Drinkaware (maintaining levels of financial support), further action on advertising and marketing (including a new sponsorship code, not advertising near schools and adhering to Drinkaware guidelines), and supporting community action to tackle alcohol harms (through local schemes such as Best Bar None and Pubwatch – see below). To persuade non-industry organizations to support the RD, concessions were offered. The RD Alcohol Network and its working groups (which would take forward specific issues such as education and retail practices) would be co-chaired by an industry and a non-industry member. Evaluation was also a major concern. To reassure on this, an RD Network subgroup on evaluation (including personnel from the DH, NGOs and the drinks industry) was established, which set out principles of evaluation in this area. As noted, the DH subsequently agreed to fund a programme of evaluation covering the RD as a whole.

The initial impact of the alcohol RD was difficult to ascertain and would not publicly emerge for some time. There were, however, early indications of dissatisfaction on the part of the DH itself. Lansley wrote to most of the main supermarket chains in May 2011 to remind them of the need to make further progress (Ahmed and Dunkley, 2011). He pointedly referred to Asda's pledge to remove alcohol displays from the foyer area of their stores, which so far had not been followed by its competitors. However, in early 2012, alcohol retailers did commit to further action and agreed to launch a campaign to raise consumers' understanding of the alcohol units in their drinks. In a further pledge, coinciding with the launch of the government's alcohol strategy in March 2012 (Cm 8336, 2012), which heralded a stronger approach (for example, on minimum pricing for alcohol and further licensing restrictions), the industry agreed to remove one billion units of alcohol from the drinks market by reducing the alcoholic content of its existing products, introducing new lower strength products and encouraging people to drink in smaller measures. Even so, this failed to impress the Health Committee (2012b) in a further report on alcohol. This identified weaknesses in the RD and was sceptical of the industry's commitment and its pledges so far. It also called on government to ensure that the RD was not a substitute for public policy, and endorsed a proper independent evaluation of this initiative.

Food

The RD food network established a core collective commitment to adopt a healthier diet. This related to three pledges: from September 2011, to provide calorie labelling on food and non-alcoholic drinks in 'out-of-home settings' (that is, restaurants and takeaways); by 2012, to reduce salt levels in food by a further 15 per cent on the targets previously set by the FSA; and by the end of 2011, to remove artificial trans-fats from food products. Although apparently substantial, these agreements did not go as far or as fast as many health campaigners had demanded. There was no deadline set for calorie labelling, for example. The target for the reduction of salt levels was unambitious, and unlikely to produce the degree of decline in salt consumption needed to reach the 6 grams a day maximum recommended level for adults. The removal of trans-fats was more radical. But, as with other collective pledges, companies did not have to sign up if they did not want to.

A number of health organizations were uneasy about the RD process and critical of business influence. There was disappointment with the weakness of the collective pledges (although it should be noted that the food pledges tended to be more systematic with deadline dates for beginning action or achievement). Two organizations expected to support the RD, Diabetes UK and the British Heart Foundation, did not sign up. Others expressed disappointment with the weakness of the pledges but nonetheless joined. Some reports suggested that health groups became increasingly disillusioned with the food aspects of the RD only months after its introduction (Ahmed and Dunkley, 2011). Evaluation of the deal confirmed some of the fears felt at the time it was launched. A report by the Children's Food Campaign (2011) found that pledges had not been universally adopted, with some large food companies adopting only one or two of the collective pledges and some not signing up at all. A number of fast-food companies refused to sign the salt reduction pledge, while some did not agree to eliminate trans-fats.

A further report on the food RD by Which? (2012) found that the attempt to secure pledges from business had been inadequate and lacked 'real leadership'. Forty-five organizations were committed to calorie labelling, but not all were providing full information for all their outlets. Furthermore, only two of the top 10 restaurant chains at this stage agreed to calorie labelling. The salt reduction pledge had 70 organizations committed to it, but this excluded many big name brands. There was more success on the removal of trans-fats, with 90 companies agreeing to this, but there was much to be done to secure agreement from small and medium-sized catering and food businesses. Which? recommended a tougher approach with stronger salt reduction targets and a robust pledge for fat and sugar reduction. It also called for the reduction of saturated fat to be a priority, with incentives and timelines introduced, a ban on trans-fats, and compulsory calorie labelling in chain restaurants. Which? called for the FSA to be given back the responsibilities for food nutrition and labelling that the Coalition government had removed in 2010, along with the implementation across the food industry of the traffic light system of food labelling. Other action demanded by Which? and others included improvements in standards of food across public institutions and commitments from food companies to ensure that foods high in fat, salt and sugar were not actively and aggressively promoted to children.

As in the case of alcohol, health campaigners feared that the government was abdicating responsibility and would not adopt a stronger approach to nutrition and obesity involving regulation and taxation. These fears were confirmed by the government's obesity strategy in autumn 2011, a low-key document that strongly emphasized self-regulation and a voluntary approach based on corporate and individual responsibility (DH, 2011e). It emphasized healthy choices, giving people information and support, and a continued emphasis on the RD. Taxation, the creation of incentives to promote healthy eating, stronger regulation and legislation, and investment in a healthier food environment did not feature. The plan was heavily criticized by health campaigners, including Jamie Oliver (2011), who branded it 'worthless, regurgitated, patronizing rubbish'. Further suspicions about the government's intentions were fuelled by the disbanding of an expert advisory committee on obesity that included critics of government policy. However, the government's strategy heralded a fourth RD pledge in this field: a reduction in total calorie consumption of five billion calories a day. Under this pledge, companies would agree to support and enable customers to eat and drink fewer calories by reformulating products and menus, reviewing portion sizes, education and information, and shifting marketing towards lower calorie options. However, this seemingly ambitious pledge was viewed as far too vague by critics (Limb, 2012; Which?, 2012).

Other parts of the RD

The other elements of the RD were much less controversial. The physical activity network established five collective pledges: getting adults and children more active; contributing to the communication and promotion of the Chief Medical Officer's physical activity guidelines; promoting and supporting active travel; increasing physical activity in the workplace; and tackling barriers to participation faced by some of most inactive groups in society. Although these were laudable aims, the commitments were very vague, and there was no mention of targets or deadlines (although the pledge on active travel included a commitment for organizations to set measurable targets in this area). The Health at Work Network was also relatively uncontroversial. It included the following pledges: managing chronic conditions at work, using new occupational health standards; including a section on employee health and well-being in annual reports and on websites; and implementing some basic measures for encouraging healthier food and drink for staff (for example, working with caterers to provide healthier meals, the provision of calories and nutrient information on staff canteen menus, and ensuring drinking water is available).

Local partnership initiatives

Current government policy favours the development of public–private partnerships (see Chapter 4). The intention is to widen the potential pool of suppliers of NHS services to include more commercial organizations and social enterprises. It should be noted that public health services (many of which have been transferred to local government) have little protection from these new competitive forces, and it is expected that a larger market for such services will develop. However, even at present there are many examples of public–private partnership working at local level on public health. Surprisingly little has been written about them, and as a result it is possible only to give a flavour of the kinds of partnership that currently exist.

Pharmacies

The potential role of community-based pharmacy businesses in promoting health has long been acknowledged. It has also been encouraged by recent governments (DH, 2005; Cm 7985, 2010). In some areas, pharmacies have developed a broader health promotion role, giving advice and support on health issues (weight management, smoking cessation and alcohol), undertaking screening and testing for diseases (such as diabetes testing, chlamydia screening, and the identification of risk factors for heart disease and stroke) and service provision (smoking cessation, contraception, vaccination and alcohol misuse and drug-related services such as needle exchange and methadone maintenance). Pharmacies can also promote the health of people not registered with a GP, often the poorest and most vulnerable section of society. This has usually occurred as a result of a proactive effort by local pharmacies and/or the local NHS. Large chains such as Boots and Lloyds Pharmacies have also been instrumental in developing local schemes and working with the NHS. However, it is also recognized that much more needs to be done to exploit the potential of such businesses in this area. The Cameron Coalition government established a working group to explore this.

Alcohol problems

With regard to the prevention of alcohol problems, businesses have attempted to build partnerships with local authorities, the police and the NHS. Schemes such as Pubwatch, Best Bar None and Nightsafe involve the licensed trade in efforts to raise standards, in conjunction with local statutory agencies (Baggott, 2006). A number of schemes have attracted national attention, including Manchester City Centre Safe (Brown and Greenacre, 2005), which sought to reduce alcohol problems related to the night-time economy and involved police working closely with the licensed trade business and local government. Another scheme, based in St Neots,

Cambridgeshire, and applauded by MPs (Culture, Media and Sport Committee, 2009), involved local police, parents, healthcare professionals and schools working together to reduce underage drinking and has since been rolled out to other towns and cities. In addition, Business Improvement Districts, where businesses pay towards improvements in the local trading environment, and Town Centre Management Initiatives have been used to target particular problems such as alcohol-related problems (for example, by providing street wardens and better management of problems related to binge drinking). Across the country, alcohol retailers have also promoted 'proof of age' schemes to prevent sales to underage drinkers (such as Challenge 21 and Challenge 25) in partnership with local agencies.

Workplace health

Workplace health is a major area of partnership working between public and private sectors. Some, particularly the larger companies, have well-established health schemes often set up with input from private healthcare providers (such as screening services and rehabilitation after injury or illness). In recent years, the emphasis has shifted away from these areas of work towards promoting health and preventing disease among the workforce. For example, BT's Work Fit programme, launched in 2005, aimed to improve nutrition and exercise among its employees. Staff received free pedometers, health information materials and a tape measure to record their waist size. They were expected to record data and were offered support from a lifestyle adviser. A follow-up survey found that most staff maintained lifestyle improvements and achieved significant weight loss. BT has also introduced initiatives on promoting mental health (IDeA, 2012).

Large companies, and public sector employers, have the resources to invest in employee health programmes, but smaller and medium-sized enterprises can benefit as well. The benefits of workplace-based health programmes were demonstrated by the Well@Work project. This project, funded by the DH, the British Heart Foundation and the National Lottery between 2005 and 2007, sought to implement a range of workplace-based health promotion interventions (such as pedometers, cycling to work schemes, health checks and healthy eating initiatives). Over 30 workplaces participated in the scheme. The evaluation found that interventions could increase physical activity and healthy diet, as well as improve staff morale (Loughborough University, 2008). However, it found significant barriers that impeded implementation, including restrictions imposed by the physical environment of the workplace, a lack of facilities and amenities, and the practical constraints of work schedules. The coordination of policies, ownership by employees and support from management was seen as essential for the success of such schemes.

The contribution of employers (both private and public) to employee health has been further underlined by government policies in recent years such as *Choosing Health* (Cm 6374, 2004), the *Strategy for Health and Well-being of Working Age People* (HM Government, 2005), the Black Review (2008) of health and work, and the Darzi Review of the NHS (Cm 7432, 2008). The key themes of all these policy documents is that more must be done to improve the health of workers and ensure that they are fit to work. In addition, the National Institute for Health and Care Excellence (previously the National Institute for Health and Clinical Excellence) has produced specific guidance on promoting health and well-being in the workplace and reducing sickness absence (NICE, 2008a, 2008b, 2009a, 2009b).

Obesity and a healthier diet

A multiagency approach involving the private sector was also a feature of anti-obesity and nutrition initiatives, The Labour government's strategy for obesity explicitly endorsed partnerships between the NHS and the private sector (HM Government, 2008a). In practice, however, the use of private sector organizations to deliver obesity interventions has been patchy. Much depends on local commissioners and pathways for managing people who are overweight and obese. Nonetheless, some companies have made inroads here. Weightwatchers (2011), for example, declared that it had weight management contracts with two-thirds of Primary Care Trusts (PCTs). Notably, there is some evidence to suggest that private weight management providers may be more effective in helping people to lose weight than conventional NHS services (Jebb et al., 2011). Some PCTs commissioned other services to help people to reduce weight through physical activity. Private gyms, alongside local authority leisure centres, are increasingly offering these services. In addition, private clubs and amenity groups, some of which are businesses and others social enterprises (see Box 7.1) or voluntary organizations, have been involved in local initiatives to encourage people to take up physical activities including cycling, walking, badminton, tennis and swimming.

The availability of healthy food is another area where the private sector has been closely involved. As already noted, under C4L, businesses were encouraged to promote and provide incentives for healthy eating. A DH-funded project under the auspices of C4L aimed to encourage convenience stores to stock and promote healthy foods. The project both improved customers' perceptions of the stores and increased the sales of fruit and vegetables (DH, 2010e). The C4L brand was also used to badge other partnership initiatives at local level to promote healthy eating. In some local areas, PCTs and local authorities have built relationships with particular businesses, such as supermarkets, to promote healthy eating messages. Community food projects have also been established to supply healthy and nutritious food to communities, often those in poverty or facing disadvantage. Although these are in many cases run by voluntary organizations, some have been established as social enterprises. These organizations work closely with private producers (farmers and small shops) to ensure their supplies (such as the Community Food Enterprise Ltd based in Newham, London; see Sustain 2005).

There are few studies of the effectiveness of such interventions. However, an analysis of one local initiative that sought to incentivize the private sector to promote healthier food and nutrition illustrated the kinds of problem encountered (Hanratty et al., 2012). Two interventions were deployed during the study period: awards for premises that provided healthy options and awards for those that welcomed breastfeeding mothers. Researchers found that the application of these policies often involved compromise (such as giving awards to businesses that had made only a minimal effort to make healthier options available), and that the awards themselves had a low profile. They also revealed that that these interventions had a low priority, both for the local public health teams and for businesses. Working with businesses was seen as a major challenge, especially in the absence of existing relationships with the sector, a lack of staff with knowledge and experience of business, and the absence of a clear national framework for businesses to become engaged in health promotion activities. Lack of time was also cited as a key obstacle.

The private sector is involved in public health initiatives in many other ways, and in some cases is an important channel for wider public health advice and support. There are many innovative cases. In Sefton, Merseyside, for example, the local PCT worked with taxi drivers to promote Men's Health. The scheme (known as 'Colin the Cabbie') used the taxi drivers as a focal point for a range of health promotion messages to passengers. The taxi drivers themselves helped to develop these materials and were engaged in activities to promote their own health, such as healthy eating and physical activity.

Conclusion

As Hunter et al. (2011) observed, those involved in public health at a local level now see the business sector as a crucial partner and have identified a need to involve it more closely in partnership working arrangements in the future. This is especially important given current policy trends towards giving private organizations a greater slice of the health service market. Hunter et al. also called for more research into partnerships involving the private sector in public health and into what lessons can be learned. This is long overdue because, as is clear from this analysis, the private sector is already extensively involved in public health policy at international, national and local levels, but there are few studies of this role.

Is private sector involvement problematic, as some suggest? Ideologically, one can oppose private sector involvement in a blanket way, but to do so would be a mistake. The private sector can contribute to improved outcomes by providing expertise or services. Moreover, it may be able to reduce harm significantly by changing its behaviour. So there is a strong case for pragmatism, providing that this is based on good-quality research and evidence. There are, however, caveats. The particular nature of private sector involvement is crucial. In some areas, the best option will be social enterprise, with profits being reinvested in services and in the community. This model is proving attractive to public organizations as an alternative to transferring services to the for-profit sector, especially where there are conflicts of interest. Social enterprise is also increasingly being adopted as a model by voluntary organizations wishing to adopt a more market-oriented approach.

A key issue is accountability. Where private 'for-profit' organizations, or social enterprises for that matter, are involved in public health initiatives, there must be transparency, openness and public accountability. There are also particular problems when dealing with industries that may profit from ill health and therefore have conflicts of interest (such as the alcohol and food industries). Here, special safeguards are required to ensure that the influence of these industries over policy formation is limited. They may of course be allowed to air their views and present evidence. But their main role should be to engage in partnership in the implementation of policy rather than its formation. Where self-regulation and voluntary agreements exist, they must be within a clear framework of targets and deadlines, with robust monitoring systems, independent representation and public accountability, and clear sanctions for non-compliance. This may be in effect an extension of state power and control over business, and objectionable to some. But, when there is a conflict, public health must take priority over commercial considerations.

8 Conclusion

Introduction

This book has shown that partnership has become a key instrument of public health and well-being. Public health is in essence a collective enterprise that requires the cooperation and collaboration of public and private sector bodies, the voluntary sector and citizens. Efforts to promote and protect public health and increase individual and social well-being will ultimately fall short if they do not foster strong mutual and reciprocal relationships. This principle is reflected in modern public health perspectives, which place great emphasis on multisectoral action and engagement with civil society (including voluntary and private sector bodies), and on the need to ensure that health and well-being are appropriately reflected in all areas of public policy.

Understanding partnerships

Concepts and frameworks

The concept of partnership between, within and across various sectors focuses attention upon what can be achieved by mutually beneficial relationships. The value of partnership as a concept has been diluted somewhat by the confusion in terminology and the fact that similar labels (for example, collaboration, cooperation and coordination) exist and are often used interchangeably. So while 'partnership' is therefore a useful term to characterize a broad field of study relevant to public health and well-being, its utility as an analytical tool is limited. It is best seen as a starting point, an umbrella for more specific models and concepts that provide better tools of analysis. As seen in Chapter 1, efforts have been made to pinpoint the crucial elements of partnership that require investigation. These include key factors that enhance or undermine partnership working. This is useful in a practical sense, providing a framework for designing partnerships and making them work better. By establishing key criteria, this approach also provides a foundation for evaluation, potentially strengthening the quality of evidence in this field.

However, these models are very limited. They are based on a rather technocratic approach that identifies certain features or practices that reflect good or bad experiences of partnership working. They are based on a simple prescription (although this is easier said than done) of promoting 'good' characteristics and discouraging 'bad' ones.

Such models tend to be based on received wisdom rather than hard evidence. Some are very static and descriptive, although, as was shown in Chapter 1, others are more dynamic and analytical. But even these lack a critical edge and fail to link to wider political questions, such as why these arrangements are being pursued and what their implications for governance and accountability are. There is of course a wider literature on governance that acknowledges the importance of collaborative processes and the reasons why partnerships have come to the fore. But few models of partnership working explicitly acknowledge this. While practical matters may prevail, and indeed are the prime concern of planners and service providers, it is essential that partnerships are designed and operated with a full acknowledgement and understanding of the processes and forces that shaped them.

Is partnership really a good thing?

The largely uncritical nature of the literature is reflected in an assumption that partnership is a jolly good thing. This tendency has been alluded to by others, including Hunter et al. (2011) and Powell and Glenndinning (2002). Its 'Mom and apple pie' status may perhaps be to some extent merited. As we have seen, there are strong and sound reasons for wishing to encourage and promote partnership in public health and other spheres of policy. But this should not blind one to situations when partnership, or a particular form of it, is inappropriate, inefficient or ineffective. There is a strong rationalist element to the study of partnership working. The reasoning goes thus: partnership working brings benefits but also problems of its own; therefore we need to secure the benefits but reduce (or, if possible, eliminate) the problems. Various instruments have been proposed to help bring this about: central edicts and guidance, reorganization and institutional changes, duties of collaboration imposed on the parties, and financial incentives and disincentives. The history of partnership working in public health (and in other policy arenas) has been a constant battle between this idealistic rational approach and the often grim realities in practice. Tales of good intentions sabotaged by territorialism, resource disputes, a silo mentality and a host of other cultural and organizational factors abound. While the desire to pursue a rational course of action to secure socially beneficial objectives is laudable, it is dangerous to build policy and practice on assumptions that all actors are rational, and that by simply removing potential barriers and obstacles, things will improve. It is probably more realistic to accept that partnership working is difficult and flawed, and that some relationships will probably never improve much, at least in the short term.

The key problem has been that partnerships are measured against an ideal that can never be achieved in practice. Indeed, the multiplicity of partnerships arguably makes it impossible to attain multiple objectives. Although some may be mutually reinforcing (pursuing similar or overlapping objectives, or building trust between partners as a platform for action on a range of issues), a partnership formed for one objective (for example, public health) might well be undermined by a partnership formed for another reason (such as economic development). In addition, intervening with the intention of strengthening partnership working can actually make things worse – for example through counterproductive restructuring, 'initiative-itis' and a 'top-down' approach that overrides or ignores local cultures and dynamics.

It is perhaps surprising that, despite the well-documented problems faced by partnerships, there remains a strong and lasting belief that they are a good thing. There is a broadly positive narrative surrounding them. Notably, the acknowledged problems of partnerships are stated more in terms of obstacles and impediments to achieving gains, rather than as disadvantages of partnership working. As noted in Chapter 1, there are indeed several possible disadvantages associated with partnerships, and it worth recapping them: partnership is not necessarily a zero-sum game, it can incur additional costs, it often involves coercion, it can lead to centralization, it can weaken accountability, and it may be carried out for ulterior reasons (for example, to control people rather than empower them). These potential drawbacks, although serious, are rarely aired to the same degree as the advantages of partnership.

But this is not necessarily a counsel of despair. Perhaps the best way forwards is to accept that partnerships are flawed arrangements. This is not to say that we should ignore the legislative, institutional and financial constraints on partnership. Rather, we should initially focus on the purpose of a specific partnership, its context and the potential partners. The focus should be on bottom-up perspectives, identifying the key issues that need to be addressed, strengthening the relationships between the partners and then identifying what needs to change in the policy environment in order to establish a framework that facilitates stronger, more acceptable and more productive partnerships in the future. This is far more likely to work than is a top-down mandated (or indeed enforced) system of partnership. The focus then moves away from ideal, rational solutions, to ways of promoting better understanding between the parties, promoting a common culture of problem-solving, and building trust, all of which have been highlighted as key factors in building partnerships that work. It is also crucial – to labour the point – that partnerships are fully evaluated and that we learn accurate lessons from them.

Evaluation and lesson-drawing

There are methodological difficulties in evaluating partnerships, as noted in Chapter 1, but they are not insurmountable. Indeed, there have been some every good studies of partnership working (notably, Hunter et al., 2011). However, there seems to have been a reluctance to evaluate, despite the existence of a number of useful frameworks. A huge amount of effort has gone into local partnership arrangements and projects, but these are rarely evaluated, and if they are, this is done crudely (focusing strongly on the impact on relationships between the partners, often in a highly subjective way, and ignoring outcomes) and/or the lessons are not communicated to a wider audience. There has been little effort to learn from experience. This not simply a UK or single-country problem but is also evident at the national and international levels. Despite partnership working in public health being an issue for all countries, there is hardly any sharing of experience and transfer of ideas and approaches. The exception perhaps is the support for partnership working from the World Health Organization and other international bodies noted in Chapter 2. But even this has been very general and predicated on a weak evidence base. Moreover, even in the UK, where one finds variations in partnership working between the different nations (see Chapters 3, 5 and 6), the opportunity for drawing lessons and learning from others' experience has not been exploited.

Why has partnership working been pursued?

One might raise questions about the motives of those who champion partnership working. Certainly, a sceptic may argue that partnership is promoted precisely because it provides a means of shifting responsibility onto others, dilutes account-ability, enables control of others, and imposes costs on them. This is not to say that partnerships are established always and everywhere for such base motives. Nor is it correct to assert that no good ever comes from partnerships, even if the reason for establishing them is cynical. Rather, it is a warning to those who take a 'rose-tinted' view of partnership, devoid of any underlying model of political power. Partnership may be more about protecting the power of governing elites, public agencies and private interests than is commonly thought. National politicians are able to shift responsibility while continuing to exert authority over local agencies (see Chapters 3 and 4); local agencies and professionals may also be able to evade responsibilities by discharging functions through partnership bodies; while private interests may avoid full responsibility by working in partnership with government (see Chapter 7). An understanding of power relationships may also explain the relative weakness of the voluntary sector in partnership arrangements (Chapter 6) and the weakness of citizen participation structures in health policy and planning (Chapter 5).

As has been noted, central government in the UK and elsewhere has been extremely active in promoting partnerships in the public health arena. These have included steps to strengthen partnership working between public agencies; and measures to form partnerships and engage with the public, the voluntary or third sector, and the private sector. There are a number of reasons why governments have intervened in this way. First, the problematization of existing partnership arrangements drew central government into a constant process of reviewing and renewing partnership structures and frameworks relevant to public health. New Labour governments, for example, were extremely active in this regard – such as in introducing Health Action Zones, Healthy Living Centres, Local Strategic Part-nerships, Local Area Agreements, Joint Strategic Needs Assessments and the volun-tary sector Compacts, and reforming patient and public involvement structures (twice). Although the Coalition government has dismantled some of its predeces-sor's work, it has demonstrated much enthusiasm for partnership working with the creation of Health and Wellbeing Boards, new place-based partnership initiatives, reformed structures for patient and public involvement and the Responsibility Deal. Second, partnership working became acknowledged as the standard response to complex social problems, to deal with so-called 'wicked issues' (see Chapter 1). Third, and related to this, wider changes in governance – the attraction of networked forms of governance, particularly in the light of welfare pluralism, the rise of the voluntary sector and privatization – favoured partnerships as a mode of governance. Fourth, partnership fitted neatly with the dominant ideological force behind all recent governments: the desire to reduce the responsibilities of central government and transfer responsibility on to others, including local government, other local agencies, the voluntary and private sectors and citizens.

The development of partnership working was not, however, simply due to top-down approaches to governance. There were pressures from below, from practitioners, from service users and from the voluntary and private sectors, to establish more effective partnership arrangements and forms of engagement. For example, the voluntary sector pressed for a greater role in service provision and policy-making. Similarly, the private sector was keen on becoming more closely involved with government, in some cases to pre-empt tougher regulation and in others to secure a share of the growing public health services market. There were also pressures towards a greater emphasis on partnership emanating from the professional sphere, encouraging cross-disciplinary and interprofessional working through the promise of more cost-effective service provision in public health.

The future

The key factors that have shaped partnership working in the past couple of decades are still with us and are likely to endure. The following will remain important: demands from service users and the public for greater accountability and more responsive services; the need to deal with service fragmentation exacerbated by greater pluralism in the supply of public services; and the persistence of public policy issues that are deemed 'wicked' and require the involvement of different agencies, sectors and the wider community (such as health inequalities, environmental health issues and obesity). One can expect further reforms of partnership arrangements, at all levels and of all types. Furthermore, I share Hunter et al.'s (2011) view that partnerships in public health are becoming more complex and that this is likely to continue.

Although this book was never intended as a manual on 'how to do partnerships' or even how to evaluate them, it nevertheless does have a practical value. Although the main purpose was to enlighten readers about the various forms of partnership in the field of public health and well-being, I also wanted to produce something that might be useful to practitioners and policy-makers. In particular, I thought it might be helpful to encourage them to reflect on the meaning of partnership, and how and when various forms of partnership might help in achieving desirable goals, such as improvements in health and well-being. So it would be remiss not to end by making a list of key recommendations based on the observations made in this book (Box 8.1).

Box 8.1	Key recommendations for partnership working

- More and better quality research is needed in this field. Evaluation of partnerships should be undertaken routinely and according to clear standards (for example, by independent researchers using acceptable methods) and criteria. Evaluation must examine the impact on outcomes as well as processes.
- Evaluation should be undertaken with the aim of sharing lessons and enabling others to learn from experience. This applies at the international, national and local levels. Those with responsibilities for public health intelligence and evidence should actively seek to collate and systematically analyse the findings from such studies.
- There must be greater consensus on the meaning of the term 'partnership' that reflects the different types and forms of collaborative working, including the private sector, voluntary sector and wider community. This does not require complete agreement on the meaning of every specific term, but at least a better understanding of what partnership means, especially among those who are involved in such arrangements.
- A more balanced approach must be taken to the value of partnership working. The potential disadvantages of partnership working must be explicitly acknowledged and given a weight equal to the potential advantages. Ways of minimizing these disadvantages should be given the same consideration as measures to realize the benefits of partnership working. Furthermore, partnership working should not be measured against an unattainable ideal but recognized as a contested area where diverse partners will negotiate potential solutions. It must also be acknowledged that there are situations where partnership working is not the best option or even a realistic one.
- It is possible to identify obstacles to effective partnership working and introduce institutional change, incentives, support and regulation to this end. This must, however, be done on the basis of research into the experiences of partnership working on the ground. It should also be noted that such interventions also have costs and may, at least in the short term, disrupt and undermine partnerships. Structural reorganization in health and local government, including the reallocation of responsibilities for public health, is a case in point.
- The power relationships underpinning various forms of partnership working must be explicitly acknowledged by all parties. Where genuine engagement is being sought, measures must be put in place to address inequitable power relations and promote accountability. Failure to do so will lead ultimately to disaffection and partnership failure. This is particularly pertinent in partnerships involving citizens and the voluntary sector.
- There must be greater acknowledgement of, and openness about, conflicts of interest in partnership working. This is particularly important where the private sector is involved, but is also relevant to the voluntary and statutory sectors.
- Greater emphasis must be placed on building partnerships from the bottom up, strengthening collaborative values, promoting a culture of engagement and building trust.
- Efforts must be undertaken to improve the public understanding of partnerships in public health. This is necessary in order to improve the visibility of partnerships, strengthen public accountability and build confidence and trust in these arrangements.
- Partnership working must be based on adequate resources and involve proactive capacity-building. Those involved in partnerships should be furnished with the necessary skills of partnership working and a broader understanding of the purpose and context of partnerships.

Bibliography

Abbot, S., Chapman, J. and Shaw, S. (2005) 'Flattening the NHS hierarchy: the case of public health', *Policy Studies*, 26(2), 133–48.

Acheson, N. (1989) *Voluntary Action and the State in Northern Ireland* (Belfast: Northern Ireland Council for Voluntary Action).

ACEVO (Association of Chief Executives of Voluntary Organizations) (2010) *The Organised Efforts of Society: The Role of the Voluntary Sector in Improving the Health of the Population* (London: ACEVO).

ACEVO (2011) *Powerful People, Responsible Society – the Report of the Commission on the Big Society* (London: ACEVO).

Adamson, D. and Bromily, R. (2008) *Community Empowerment in Practice: Lessons from Communities First* (York: Joseph Rowntree Foundation).

Addicott, R. (2011) *Social Enterprise in Health Care* (London: King's Fund).

Ahmed, K. and Dunkley, J. (2011) 'Health Secretary Andrew Lansley demands supermarkets take action on alcohol', *Daily Telegraph*, 28 May 2011 (www.telegraph.co.uk; accessed 31 May 2011).

Alcock, P. (2010) 'A strategic unity: defining the third sector in the UK', *Voluntary Sector Review*, 19(1), 5–24.

Alcock, P. (2011) 'Voluntary action, New Labour and the Third Sector'. In Hilton, M. and McKay, J. (eds) *The Ages of Voluntarism* (Oxford: Oxford University Press), pp. 158–79.

Alcock, P. (2012) 'New policy spaces: the impact of devolution on third sector policy in the UK', *Social Policy and Administration*, 46(2), 219–38.

Aldridge, N. (2005) *Communities in Control: The New Third Sector Agenda for Public Service Reform*. (London: Social Market Foundation).

Allen, P., Townsend, J., Dempster, P., Wright, J., Hutchings, A. and Keen, J. (2012) 'Organisational form as a mechanism to involve staff, public users in public services: a study of the governance of foundation trusts', *Social Policy and Administration*, 46(3), 239–57.

Allin, S., Mossialos, E., McKee, M. and Holland, W. (2004) *Making Decisions on Public Health: A Review of Eight Countries* (Copenhagen: WHO/European Observatory on Health Systems and Policies).

Almedom, A. (2005) 'Social capital and mental health: an interdisciplinary review of primary evidence', *Social Science and Medicine*, 61, 943–64.

Amos, M. (2002) 'Community development'. In Adams, L., Amos, M. and Munro, J. (eds) *Promoting Health: Politics and Practice* (London: Sage), pp. 63–71.

Antonovsky, A. (1979) *Health, Stress and Coping* (San Francisco: Jossey-Bass).

Antonovsky, A. (1996) 'The salutogenic model as a theory to guide health promotion', *Health Promotion International*, 11(1), 11–18.

Arie, S. (2011) 'How should GAVI build on its success?', *BMJ*, 343, d5182, 8 September (accessed 31 May 2012).

Armingeon, K. and Beyeler, M. (2004) *The OECD and European Welfare States* (Cheltenham: Edward Elgar).

Arnstein, S. (1969) 'A ladder of citizen participation in the USA', *American Institute of Planners Journal*, 35, 216–24.

Ashton, J. (ed.) (1992) *Healthy Cities* (Milton Keynes: Open University).

Audit Commission (1998) *Effective Partnership Working* (London: Audit Commission).

Audit Commission (2005) *A Fruitful Partnership: Effective Partnership Working* (London: Audit Commission).

Audit Commission (2007a) *Improving Health and Well-being* (London: Audit Commission).

Audit Commission (2007b) *Hearts and Minds: Commissioning from the Third Sector* (London: TSO).

Audit Commission (2008) *Are We There Yet? Improving Governance and Resource Management in Children's Trusts* (London: Audit Commission).

Audit Commission (2009) *Working Better Together: Managing Local Strategic Partnerships* (London: Audit Commission).

Audit Commission (2010a) *Healthy Balance* (London: Audit Commission).

Audit Commission (2010b) *Giving Children a Healthy Start* (London: Audit Commission).

Audit Scotland (2011) *Review of Community Health Partnerships* (Edinburgh: Audit Scotland).

Audit Scotland (2013) *Improving Community Planning in Scotland* (Edinburgh, Audit Scotland).

Australian Government (2009) *Australia: The Healthiest Country by 2020. National Preventative Health Strategy Overview* (Canberra: Australian Government).

Australian Government (2010) 'Taking preventive action. A response to Australia: the healthiest country by 2020 – the report of the National Preventative Task Force' (www.preventativehealth.org.au/internet/preventativehealth/publishing.nsf/Content/6B7B17659424FBE5CA257720 00095458/$File/tpa.pdf; accessed 15 May 2013).

Babor, T., Caetano, R., Casswell, S., Edwards, G., Giesbrecht, N., Graham, K. et al. (2003) *Alcohol: No Ordinary Commodity. Research and Public Policy* (Oxford: Oxford University Press).

Bache, I. and Flinders, M. (eds) (2004) *Multi-level Governance* (Oxford: Oxford University Press).

Baggott, R. (1986) 'By voluntary agreement: the politics of instrument selection', *Public Administration*, 64(1), 51–69.

Baggott, R. (1989) 'Regulatory reform in Britain: the changing face of self regulation', *Public Administration*, 67, 435–54.

Baggott, R. (1990) *Alcohol, Politics and Social Policy* (Aldershot: Avebury).

Baggott, R. (2005) 'A funny thing happened on the way to the forum? Reforming patient and public involvement in the NHS in England', *Public Administration*, 83(3), 533–51.

Baggott, R. (2006) *Alcohol Strategy and the Drinks Industry: A Partnership for Prevention?* (York: York Publishing Services).

Baggott, R. (2010a) *Public Health: Policy and Politics* (2nd edn) (Basingstoke: Palgrave).

Baggott, R. (2010b) 'Alcohol policy and New Labour: a modern approach to an old problem?', *Policy and Politics*, 38(1), 135–52.

Baggott, R. and Jones, K. (2011) 'Prevention better than cure?: health consumer and patients' organisations and public health', *Social Science and Medicine*, 73(4), 530–4.

Baggott, R., Allsop, J. and Jones, K. (2005) *Speaking for Patients and Carers: Health Consumer Groups and the Policy Process* (Basingstoke: Palgrave).

Bakan, S. (2005) *The Corporation: The Pathological Pursuit of Profit and Power* (London: Constable).

Ball, J. and Pike, G. (2005) *Results from a Census Survey of RCN School Nurses* (London: RCN).

Ball, R., Forbes, T., Parris, M. and Forsyth, L. (2010) 'The evaluation of partnership working in the delivery of health and social care', *Public Policy and Administration*, 25(4), 387–407.

Balloch, S. and Taylor, M. (2001) *Partnership Working: Policy and Practice* (Bristol: Policy Press).

Bang, H. (2005) 'Among everyday makers and expert citizens'. In Newman, J. (ed.) *Remaking Governance: Peoples, Politics and the Public Sphere* (Bristol: Policy Press), pp. 157–79.

Barnard, M., Becker, E., Creegan, C., Day, N., Devitt, K., Fuller, E. et al. (2009) *Evaluation of the National Healthy Schools Programme Interim Report* (London: National Centre for Social Research).

Barnes, M., Bauld, L., Benzeval, M., Judge, K., Mackenzie, M. and Sullivan, H. (2005) *Health Action Zones: Partnerships for Health Equity* (London: Routledge).

Barnes, M., Newman, J. and Sullivan, H. (2007) *Power, Participation and Political Renewal* (Bristol: Policy Press).

Batniji, R. and Woods, N. (2009) *Averting a Crisis for Global Health: 3 Actions for the G20* (Oxford: Global Economic Governance Programme).

Batt, S. (1994) *Patient No More: The Politics of Breast Cancer* (London: Scarlett Press).

Bauld, L. and McKenzie, M. (2007) 'Health action zones: multi-agency partnerships to improve health'. In Scriven, A. and Garman, S. (eds) *Public Health: Social Context and Action* (Basingstoke: Palgrave), pp. 131–43.

Baum, F. (2002) *The New Public Health* (2nd edn) (Oxford: Oxford University Press).

Beecham Review (2006) *Beyond Boundaries: Citizen-centred Local Services for Wales. Review of Local Service Delivery*. Report to the Welsh Assembly Government. (Cardiff: WAG).

Belsky, J., Melhuish, E., Barnes, J., Leyland, A. and Romaniuk, H. (2006) 'Effects of Sure Start local programmes on children and families: early findings from a quasi-experimental, cross sectional study', *BMJ*, 332, 1476–78.

Berlinguer, G. (1999) 'Globalisation and global health', *International Journal of Health Services*, 29(3), 579–95.

Berridge, V. (1996) *AIDS in the UK: The Making of Policy 1981–1994* (Oxford University Press).

Better Regulation Task Force (1998) *Access to Government Funding for the Voluntary and Community Sector* (London: Better Regulation Task Force).

Better Regulation Task Force (1999) *Self-regulation: Interim Report* (London: Better Regulation Task Force).

Better Regulation Task Force (2005) *Better Regulation for Civil Society: Making Life Easier for Those Who Help Others* (London: Better Regulation Task Force).

Black, C. (2008) *Working for a Healthier Tomorrow: Dame Carol Black's Review of the Health of Britain's Working Age Population* (London: TSO).

Blaug, R. (2002) 'Engineering democracy', *Political Studies*, 50, 102–16.

Blond, P. (2010) *Red Tory: How Left and Right Have Broken Britain and How We Can Fix It* (London: Faber).

BMA (British Medical Association) (2009) *Under the Influence: The Damaging Effect of Alcohol Marketing on Young People* (London: BMA).

Bonell, A., McKee, M., Fletcher, A., Wilkinson, P. and Haines, A. (2011) 'One nudge forwards two steps back', *BMJ*, 342, d401, 25 January (accessed 14 September 2011).

Bonell, C., Hargreaves, J., Cousens, S., Ross, D., Hayes, R., Petticrew, M. et al. (2011) 'Alternatives to randomisation in the evaluation of public health interventions; design challenges and solutions', *Journal of Epidemiology and Community Health*, 65(7), 582–7.

Borgonovi, F. (2010) 'A lifecycle approach to the analysis of the relationship between social capital and health', *Social Science and Medicine*, 71, 1927–34.

Boseley, S., Ball, J. and Syal, R. (2011) 'Coalition policy in tatters as health experts rebel', *Guardian*, 17 February, p. 1.

Bowles, M. (2010) *The Current Context for Community Development*. Independent Expert Panel on Community Development Panel Paper 1 (www.cdx.org.uk; accessed 8 May 2012).

Boyd, A. and Coleman, A. (2011) 'Strategies used by health scrutiny committees to influence decision makers', *Local Government Studies*, 37(3), 253–74.

Boydell, L. and Rugkåsa, J. (2007) 'Benefits of working in partnership: a model', *Critical Public Health*, 17, 217–28.

Boydell, L., Hoggett, P., Rugkasa, J. and Cummins, A.-M. (2008) 'Intersectoral partnerships, the knowledge economy and intangible assets', *Policy and Politics*, 36(2), 209–24.

Boyle, D. and Harris, M. (2009) *The Challenge of Co-production* (London: New Economics Foundation/NESTA).

Briggs, A. (1959) *The Age of Improvement* (London: Longman).

Bromley By Bow Centre (2012) www.bbbc.org.uk/pages/history-of-the-centre.html (accessed 13 December 2012).

Brown, B. and Liddle, B. (2005) 'Service domains – the new communities: a case study of Peterlee Sure Start UK', *Local Government Studies*, 31(4), 449–73.

Brown, J. and Greenacre, S. (2005) 'Manchester City Centre Safe: a demonstration project'. In Kolvin, P. (ed.) *Licensed Premises: Law and Practice* (Haywards Heath: Tottel), pp. 702–30.

Brown, P., Mayer, B., Zavestoski, S., Luebke, T., Mandelbaum, J. and McCormick, S. (2003) 'The health politics of asthma: environmental justice and collective illness experience in the United States', *Social Science and Medicine*, 57, 453–64.

Brugha, R. and Walt, G. (2011) 'A global health fund: a leap of faith', *BMJ*, 323, 152–4.

Buck, D. and Frosini, F. (2012) *Clustering of Unhealthy Behaviours over Time: Implications for Policy and Practice* (London: King's Fund).

Bull, M. (2008) 'Challenging tensions: critical, theoretical and empirical perspectives on social enterprise', Guest Editorial, *International Journal of Entrepreneurial Behaviour & Research*, 14(5), 268–75.

Burke, E. (1987) *Reflection on the Revolution in France* (New York: Prometheus).

Burton, P., Croft, J., Hastings, A., Slater, T., Goodlad, R., Abbott, J. et al. (2008) *What Works in Community Involvement in Area Based Initiatives? A Systematic Review of the Literature* (London: Home Office).

Buse, K. and Harmer, A. (2007) 'Seven habits of highly effective global public-private health partnerships: practice and potential', *Social Science and Medicine*, 64, 259–71.

Buse, K. and Walt, G. (2000) 'Global-public health partnerships. Part 2. What are the issues for global governance?', *Bulletin of the World Health Organization*, 78(5), 699–709.

Buse, K. and Waxman, A. (2001) 'Public-private partnerships: a strategy for WHO', *Bulletin of the World Health Organization,* 79(8), 748–54.

Butterfoss, F. (2007) *Coalitions and Partnerships in Community Health* (San Francisco: Jossey Bass).

Butterfoss, F., Goodman, R. and Wandersman, A. (1993) 'Community coalitions for prevention and health promotion', *Health Education Research*, 8(3), 315–30.

Byrne, D. (2004) *Partnership for Health in Europe* (Brussels: European Commission).

Cabinet Office (2002) *Strategy Unit Report: Private Action, Public Benefit. A Review of Charities and the Wider Not-For-Profit Sector* (London: Cabinet Office).

Cabinet Office (2007) *Capability Review of the Department of Health* (London: Cabinet Office).

Cabinet Office (2010) *Building the Big Society* (London: Cabinet Office).

Caines, K. (2004) *Global Health Partnerships: Assessing the Impact* (London: Department for International Development).

Cairney, P., Studlar, D. and Mamudu, H. (2012) *Global Tobacco Control* (Basingstoke: Palgrave).

Cairns, B., Harris, M. and Hutchinson, R. (2006) *Servants of the Community or Agents of Government?* (London: IVAR).

Calkin, S. (2013) 'Local healthwatch will be bound and gagged', *Health Service Journal*, 17 January, 13.

Campbell, D. (2012) 'Doctors dismayed as public health committee is scrapped', *The Guardian On line*, 8 December (www.guardian.co.uk; accessed 17 January 2013).

Cameron, A. and Lart, R. (2003) 'Factors promoting and obstacles hindering joint working: a systematic review of the research evidence', *Journal of Integrated Care*, 11(2), 9–17.

Canadian Institutes for Health Research (2003) *The Future of Public Health in Canada; Developing a Public Health System for the 21st Century* (Ottawa: Canadian Institutes of Health Research).

Cannon, G. (1987) *The Politics of Food* (London: Century Hutchinson).

Carmel, E. and Harlock, J. (2008) 'Instituting the "third sector" as a governable terrain: partnership, procurement and performance in the UK', *Policy and Politics*, 36(2), 155–71.

Carroll, A. (1999) 'Corporate social responsibility: evolution of a definitional construct', *Business and Society*, 38(3), 268–95.

Carter, N. (2007) *The Politics of the Environment: Ideas, Activism, Policy* (2nd edn) (Cambridge: Cambridge University Press).

Castell-Florit, P. (2010) 'Intersectoral health strategies: from discourse to action', *MEDICC Review*, 12(1), 48.

Cattell, V. (2001) 'Poor people, poor places and poor health: the mediating role of social networks and social capital', *Social Science and Medicine*, 52, 1501–46.

Cd 4499 (1909) *Royal Commission on the Poor Laws and Relief of Distress*, Majority and Minority Report (London: HMSO).

Celia, C., Diepeveen, S. and Ling, T. (2010) *The European Alcohol and Health Forum: First Monitoring Progress Report* (Cambridge: Rand Europe).

Centre for Public Scrutiny (2011) *Smoothing the Way: Developing Local Healthwatch Through Lessons from Local Involvement Networks* (London: CPS).

Challis, L., Fuller, S., Henwood, M., Klein, R., Plowden, W., Webb, A. et al. (1988) *Joint Approaches to Social Policy* (Cambridge: Cambridge University Press).

Chapman, J., Shaw, S., Congdon, P., Carter, Y., Abbott, S. and Petchey, R. (2005) 'Specialist public health capacity in England: working in the new primary care organisations', *Public Health*, 119, 22–31.

Charities Aid Foundation/NCVO (2010) *UK Giving 2010* (West Malling: Charities Aid Foundation).

Charity Commission (2008) *CC9 – Speaking Out – Guidance on Campaigning and Political Activity by Charities* (London: Charity Commission).

Charles, C. and De Maio, S. (1993) 'Lay participation in healthcare decision making: a conceptual framework', *Journal of Health Politics, Policy and Law*, 18, 881–904.

Children, School and Families Committee (2010) *Sure Start Children's Centres. 5th Report 2009–10*. HC 130 (London, TSO).

Children's Food Campaign (2011) *The Irresponsibility Deal* (London: Children's Food Campaign).

Churchill, N. (ed.) (2012) *Getting Started: Prospects for Health and Wellbeing Boards* (London: Smith Institute/ACCA).

Clark, J., Kane, D., Wilding, K. and Wilton, J. (2010) *UK Civil Society Almanac 2010* (London: NCVO).

Clarke, J. and Glendinning, C. (2002) 'Partnership and the remaking of welfare governance'. In Glendinning, C., Powell, M. and Rummery, K. (eds) *Partnerships, New Labour and Governance* (Bristol: Policy Press), pp. 33–50.

Clarke, J. and Newman, J. (1997) *The Managerial State* (London: Sage).

Clarke, J., Newman, J., Smith, N., Vidler, E., Vidler, E. and Westmarland, L. (2007) *Creating Citizen Consumers: Changing Public and Changing Public Services* (London: Sage).

Clark, J., McHugh, J. and McKay, S. (2011) *UK Voluntary Sector Workforce Almanac 2011* (Sheffield: Skills–Third Sector).

Clarke, M. and Stewart, J. (1997) *Handling the Wicked Issues: A Challenge for Government* (Birmingham: University of Birmingham).

Cm 249 (1987) *Promoting Better Health* (London: HMSO).

Cm 289 (1988) *Public Health in England* (London: HMSO).

Cm 555 (1989) *Working for Patients* (London: HMSO).

Cm 1986 (1992) *The Health of the Nation: A Strategy for Health in England* (London: TSO).

Cm 4100 (1998) *Compact on Relations Between Government and the Voluntary and Community Sector in England* (London: TSO).

Cm 4269 (1999) *Towards A Healthier Scotland. Scottish White Paper* (London: TSO).

Cm 4310 (1999) *Modernising Government* (London: TSO).

Cm 4386 (1999) *Saving Lives: Our Healthier Nation* (London: TSO).

Cm 4818 (2000) *The NHS Plan: A Plan for Investment – A Plan for Reform* (London: TSO).

Cm 4911 (2000) *Our Towns and Cities: The Future: Delivering an Urban Renaissance* (London: TSO).

Cm 5730 (2003) *The Victoria Climbié Inquiry: Report of an Inquiry by Lord Laming* (London: TSO).

Cm 5860 (2003) *Every Child Matters: Green Paper* (London: TSO).

Cm 6079 (2003) *Building on the Best: Choice, Responsiveness and Equity in the NHS* (London: TSO).

Cm 6374 (2004) *Choosing Health: Making Healthy Choices Easier* (London: TSO).

Cm 6737 (2006) *Our Health, Our Care, Our Say: A New Direction for Community Services* (London: TSO).

Cm 6939 (2006) *Strong and Prosperous Communities: The Local Government White Paper* (London: TSO).

Cm 7189 (2007) *The Future Role of the Third Sector in Social and Economic Regeneration: Final Report* (London: TSO).

Cm 7280 (2007) *The Children's Plan: Building Brighter Futures* (London: TSO).

Cm 7427 (2008) *Communities in Control: Real People, Real Power* (London: TSO).

Cm 7432 (2008) *High Quality Healthcare for All* (London: TSO).

Cm 7881 (2010) *Equity and Excellence: Liberating the NHS* (London: TSO).

Cm 7985 (2010) *Healthy Lives, Healthy People* (London: TSO).

Cm 8145 (2011) *Open Public Services White Paper* (London: TSO).

Cm 8290 (2012) *Response to the House of Commons Health Committee Report on Public Health* (London: TSO).

Cm 8336 (2012) *The Government's Alcohol Strategy* (London: TSO).

Cmd 693 (1920) *Interim Report on the Future Provision of Medical and Allied Services* (The Dawson Report) (London: HMSO).

Cmd 9663 (1956) *Report of the Committee of Inquiry into the Cost of the National Health Service* (The Guillebaud Report) (London: HMSO).

Cmnd 4040 (1969a) *Royal Commission on Local Government in England 1966–69. Volume I – Report* (The Redcliffe–Maud Report) (London: HMSO).

Cmnd 4040 (1969b) *Royal Commission on Local Government in England 1966–69. Volume II – Memorandum of Dissent by Mr Derek Senior* (London: HMSO).

Cmnd 7047 (1977) *Prevention and Health* (London: HMSO).

Cmnd 9716 (1986) *Report of the Committee of Inquiry into an Outbreak of Food Poisoning at Stanley Royal Hospital Wakefield* (London: HMSO).

Cmnd 9772 (1986) *First Report of the Committee of Inquiry into the Outbreak of Legionnaire's Disease in Stafford, April 1985* (London: HMSO).

Cohen, D. and Carter, P. (2010) 'WHO and the pandemic flu "conspiracies"', *BMJ*, 340, c2912, 4 June (accessed 29 September 2009).

Coleman, A. and Glendinning, C. (2004) 'Local authority scrutiny of health: making the views of the community count', *Health Expectations*, 7, 29–39.

Collin, J. and Lee, K. (2007) 'Globalisation and public health policy'. In Scriven, A. and Garman, S. (eds) *Public Health: Social Context and Action* (Maidenhead: Open University Press), pp. 105–18.

Commission of the European Communities (2007) *White Paper. Together for Health: A Strategic Approach for the EU 2008–2013*. Com 2007 630 final (Brussels: European Commission).

Commission on the Future of the Voluntary Sector (1996) *Meeting the Challenge of Change: Voluntary Action into the 21st Century: The Report of the Commission on the Future of the Voluntary Sector* (The Deakin Report) (London: NCVO).

Committee on Voluntary Organisations (1978) *The Future of Voluntary Organisations: Report of the Wolfenden Committee* (London: Croom Helm).

Commonwealth Department of Human Services and Health (1994) *Better Health Outcomes for Australians: National Goals, Targets and Strategies for Better Health Outcomes into the Next Century* (Canberra: Australian Government Publishing Service).

Communication from the Commission (2010) to the European Parliament, the Council, the European Economic and Social Committee and the Committee of the Regions. *The CAP Towards 2020. Meeting the Food, Natural Resources and Territorial Challenges of the Future.* COM 2010 672 Final, 18 November 2010.

Communities and Local Government Committee (2013) *The Role of Local Authorities in Health Issues, 8th Report 2012–13* (London: TSO).

Compact Voice (2012) *Informing and Influencing the New Local Health Landscape: A Guide for Local Compacts* (London: Compact Voice).

Compact Voice/Commission on the Compact/Local Government Association/Cabinet Office (Office of the Third Sector) (2009) *The Compact* (London: Commission for the Compact).

Conflicts of Interest Coalition (2011) 'Statement of concern' (www.babymilkaction.org; accessed 4 April 2012).

Connelly J., McAveary, M. and Griffiths, S. (2005) 'National survey of working life after Shifting the Balance of Power', *Public Health*, 119(12), 1133–77.

Conservative Party (2007) *NHS Autonomy and Accountability: Proposals for Legislation* (London: Conservative Party).

Conservative Party (2008*) Final Report of the Conservative Party Working Group on Responsible Business: A Light but Effective Touch* (London: Conservative Party).

Conservative Party (2009) *Renewal: Plan for a Better NHS* (London: Conservative Party).

Conservative Party (2010a) *Invitation to Join the Government of Britain*. Conservative General Election Manifesto 2010 (London: Conservative Party).

Conservative Party (2010b) *A Healthier Nation*. Policy Green Paper No. 12 (London: Conservative Party).

Conservative Research Department (2007) *Public Health: Our Priority* (London: Conservative Party).

Cook, D. (2002) 'Consultation, for a change? Engaging users and communities in the policy process', *Social Policy and Administration*, 36(5): 516–31.

Cooper, L., Coote, A., Davies, A. and Jackson, C. (1995) *Voices Off: Tackling the Democratic Deficit in Health* (London: IPPR).

Corbett, S. and Walker, A. (2012) 'The Big Society: back to the future', *Political Quarterly*, 83(3), 487–93.

Corporate Accountability International (2011) *Global Civil Society Groups Call on WHO, UN to Protect Water and Reject Corporate Conflicts of Interests*. Press release (www.stopcorporateabuse.org/press-release/civil-society-who-un-reject-corporate-conflict-interest; accessed 5 June, 2013).

Coulter, A. (2009) *Engaging Communities in Health Improvement: A Scoping Study for the Health Foundation* (London: Health Foundation).

Council of Europe (2000) *Recommendation R (2000) 5 of the Committee of Ministers of the Council of Europe to its Member States on the Developments of Structures for Citizen and Patient Participation in the Decision-making Process Affecting Health Care 24 February 2000.* 699th meeting of Ministers' deputies.

Council of the European Union (2010) *Council Conclusions on the EU Role in Global Health.* 3011th Foreign Affairs Council Meeting, Brussels, 10 May 2010.

Cousens, S., Hargreaves, J., Bonell, C., Armstrong, B., Thomas, J., Kirkwood, B. et al. (2011) 'Alternatives to randomisation in the evaluation of public health interventions: statistical analysis and causal inference', *Journal of Epidemiology and Community Health*, 65(7), 576–81.

Coussins, J. (2004) 'The Portman Group does not represent alcohol industry', *BMJ*, 329, 404.

CPPIH (Commission for Patient and Public Involvement in Health) (2008) *Commission for Patient and Public Involvement in Health: Report and Accounts 2007/8* (London: CPPIH).

Craig, G. and Taylor, M. (2002) 'Dangerous liaisons'. In Glendinning, C., Powell, M. and Rummery, K. (eds) *Partnerships, New Labour and the Governance of Welfare* (Bristol: Policy Press), pp. 131–47.

Craig, G., Taylor, M., Bloor, K., Wilkinson, M., Syed, A. and Munro, S. (2002) *Contract or Trust? The Role of Compacts in Local Governance* (Bristol, Policy Press).

Craig, P., Dieppe, P., Macintyre, S., Michie S., Nazareth I. and Petticrew, M. (2008) 'Developing and evaluating complex interventions: the new Medical Research Council guidance', *BMJ*, 337 a1656, 22 October (accessed 25 January 2012).

Crawshaw, P., Bunton, R. and Gillen, K. (2003) 'Health action zones and the problem of community', *Health and Social Care in the Community*, 11(1), 36–44.

Crisp, N. (2007) *Global Health Partnerships* (London, COI).

Culture, Media and Sport Committee (2009) *The Licensing Act 2003. 6th Report 2008–9.* HC 492 (London: TSO).

Curry, N., Mundle, C., Sheil, F. and Weaks, L. (2011) *The Voluntary and Community Sector in Health: Implications of the Proposed NHS Reforms* (London: King's Fund).

Daley, D. (2008) 'Interdisciplinary problems and agency boundaries: exploring effective cross agency collaboration', *Journal of Public Administration, Research and Theory*, 19(3), 477–93.

Darlow, A., Percy-Smith, J. and Wells, P. (2007) 'Community strategies: are they delivering joined up governance?', *Local Government Studies*, 33(1), 117–29.

Davidson, S. (1998) 'Spinning the wheel of empowerment', *Planning*, April, 14–15.

Davies, J. (2009) 'The limits of joined up government: towards a political analysis', *Public Administration*, 87(1), 80–96.

Davies, J. (2011) *Challenging Governance Theory: From Networks to Hegemony* (Bristol: Policy Press).

Davies, J. (2012) 'Active citizenship: navigating the conservative heartlands of the New Labour project', *Policy and Politics*, 40(1), 3–19.

Davies, J. and Kelly, M. (1992) *Healthy Cities* (Buckingham: Open University Press).

Daykin, N., Evans, D., Petsoulas, C. and Sayers, A. (2007) 'Evaluating the impact of patient and public involvement initiatives on UK health services: a systematic review', *Evidence and Policy*, 3(1), 47–65.

DCLG (Department of Communities and Local Government) (2008) *Process Evaluation of Plan Rationalisation: Formative Evaluation of Community Strategies* (London: DCLG).

DCLG (2009) *Long Term Evaluation of Local Area Agreements and Local Strategic Partnerships: Report on the 2008 Survey* (London: DCLG).

DCLG (2011a) *Long Term Evaluation of Local Area Agreements and Local Strategic Partnerships 2007–10. Final Report* (London: DCLG).

DCLG (2011b) *Citizenship Survey 2010–11* (London: DCLG).

Deakin, N. and Davis Smith, J. (2011) 'Labour, charity and voluntary action; the myths of hostility'. In Hilton, M. and McKay, J. (eds) *The Ages of Voluntarism* (Oxford: Oxford University Press), pp. 69–93.

Decision of the European Parliament and of the Council (2002) 'Decision No. 1786/2002/EC of the European Parliament and of the Council of 23 September 2002 adopting a programme of community action in the field of public health (2003–2008)', *Official Journal L 271*, 9 October 2002.

Decision of the European Parliament and of the Council (2007) 'Decision No. 1350/2007/EC of the European Parliament and of the Council of 23 October 2007 establishing a second programme of community action in the field of health (2008–13)', *Official Journal L 30*, 20 November 2007.

Department for Children, Schools and Families and DH (2009) *Healthy Lives, Brighter Futures: The Strategy for Children and Young People's Health* (London: DH).

Department of Trade and Industry (2002) *Social Enterprise: A Strategy for Success* (London: DTI).

Derrett, C. and Burke, L. (2006) 'The future of primary care nurses and health visitors', *BMJ*, 333, 1185–6.

De Vos, P., Dewitte, H. and Van der Stuyft, P. (2004) 'Unhealthy European policy', *International Journal of Health Services*, 34(2), 255–69.

De Vos, P. (2005) '"No one left abandoned": Cuba's national health system since the 1959 revolution', *International Journal of Health Services*, 35, 189–207.

DH (Department of Health) (1993) *Working Together for Better Health* (London: DH).

DH (1998a) *The Health of the Nation: A Policy Assessed* (London: TSO).

DH (1998b) *Partnership in Action: New Opportunities for Joint Working between Health and Social Services: A Discussion Document* (London: DH).

DH (1998c) *Modernising Health and Social Services: National Priorities Guidance 1999–2000/2001–2* (London: DH).

DH (1999) *Patient and Public Involvement in the New NHS* (London: DH).

DH (2001) *Report of the Chief Medical Officer's Project to Strengthen the Public Health Function* (London: DH).

DH (2003) *Tackling Health Inequalities: Programme for Action* (London: DH).

DH (2004) *Making Partnership Work for Patients, Carers and Service Users: Strategic Agreement between the Department of Health, the NHS and the Voluntary and Community Sector* (London: DH).

DH (2005) *Choosing Health Through Pharmacy: A Programme for Pharmaceutical Public Health* (London; DH).

DH (2006a) *Standards for Better Health* (London: DH).

DH (2006b) *No Excuses. Embrace Partnership Now. Step Towards Change! Report of the Third Sector Commissioning Task Force* (London: DH).

DH (2007a) *Partnerships for Better Health* (London: DH).

DH (2007b) *World Class Commissioning: Vision* (London: DH).

DH (2007c) *Commissioning Framework for Health and Wellbeing* (London: DH).

DH (2008) *A High Quality Workforce: NHS Next Stage Review* (London: DH).

DH (2010a) *Monitoring Mortality Bulletin – Infant Mortality Inequalities* (London: TSO).

DH (2010b) *Liberating the NHS: Developing the Healthcare Workforce* (London: DH).

DH (2010c) *The NHS Constitution for England* (London: DH).

DH (2010d) *Change4Life: One Year On* (London: DH).

DH (2010e) *Change4Life: Convenience Stores Evaluation Report* (London: DH).

DH (2011a) *Monitoring Mortality Bulletin* (London: TSO).

DH (2011b) *NHS Operating Framework 2012/13* (London: DH).

DH (2011c) *LINKs Annual Reports 2010–11* (London: DH).

DH (2011d) *The Public Health Responsibility Deal* (London: DH).

DH (2011e) *Healthy Lives, Healthy People: A Call to Action on Obesity* (London: DH).

DH (2011f) *Monitoring Mortality Bulletin – Infant Mortality Inequalities* (London, TSO).

DH (2012a) *The Mandate: A Mandate from the Government to the NHS Commissioning Board April 2013 to March 2015* (London: DH).

DH (2012b) *Joint Strategic Needs Assessment and Joint Health and Wellbeing Strategies – Draft Guidance* (London: DH).

DH (2012c) *Healthy Lives, Healthy People: Towards a Workforce Strategy for the Public Health Services* (London: DH/LGA).

DH (2012d) *The NHS Constitution for England* (London: DH).

DH (2012e) *Health Emergency Preparedness, Resilience and Response from April 2013* (London: DH).

DH (2013a) *Statutory Guidance on Joint Strategic Needs Assessments and Joint Health and Wellbeing Strategies* (London: DH).

DH (2013b) *Local Involvement Networks (LINKs) Annual Reports 2011–12* (London: DH).

DH/Public Health England/LGA (2013) *Healthy Lives, Healthy People: A Public Workforce Strategy* (London: DH).

DHSS (Department of Health and Social Security) (1981) *Care in Action* (London: DHSS).

DHSS (1985) *Working Group on Joint Planning Progress in Partnership* (London: DHSS).

DHSSNI (Department of Health and Social Security for Northern Ireland) (1996) *Health and Well-being Towards the New Millenium* (Belfast: DHSSNI).

DHSSNI (1997) *Well in 2000* (Belfast: DHSSNI).

DHSSPS (Department of Health Social Security and Public Safety) (2002) *Investing for Health* (Belfast: DHSSPS).

DHSSPS (2004) *Investing for Health Update* (Belfast: DHSSPS).

Douglas, R. (1998) 'A framework for healthy alliances'. In Scriven, A. (ed.) *Alliances in Health Promotion: Theory and Practice* (Basingstoke: Palgrave), pp. 3–17.

Dowling, B., Powell, M. and Glendinning, C. (2004) 'Conceptualising successful partnerships', *Health and Social Care in the Community*, 12(4), 309–17.

Driver, S. and Martell, L. (2002) *Blair's Britain* (Cambridge: Polity Press).

Earle, S. (2007) 'Promoting health in a global context'. In Lloyd, C., Handsley, S., Douglas, J., Earle, S. and Spurr, S. (2007) *Policy and Practice in Promoting Public Health* (London: Sage/Open University), pp. 1–32.

Edwards, G., West, R., Babor, T., Hall, W. and Marsden, J. (2004) 'An invitation to the alcohol industry lobby to help decide public funding of alcohol research and professional training: a decision that should be reversed', *Addiction*, 99(10), 1235–6.

El Ansari, W., Phillips, C. and Hammick, M. (2001) 'Collaboration and partnerships: developing the evidence base', *Health and Social Care in the Community*, 9(4), 215–27.

Elinder, L., Joosens, L. and Raw, M. (2003) *Public Health Aspects of the Common Agricultural Policy* (Ostersund: Swedish National Institute of Public Health).

Elkins, T. (2012) *Government and the Voluntary Sector: Investigating Funding and Engagement* (London: Compact Voice).

Elliott, L. (2004) *The Global Politics of the Environment* (London: Palgrave Macmillan).

Entwhistle, T. (2006) 'The distinctiveness of the Welsh partnership agenda', *International Journal of Public Sector Management*, 19(3), 228–37.

Eriksson, K. (2012) 'Self service society: participative politics and new forms of governance', *Public Administration*, 90(3), 685–98.

Etzioni, A. (1993) *The Spirit of Community* (New York: Random House).

EU Health Policy Forum (2007) *Guiding Principles with Regard to Transparency* (Brussels: EUHPF).

EU Ministerial Conference (2007) *Rome Declaration: Health in All Policies – Achievements and Challenges*. 18 December, Rome.

European Union (1997) *The Treaty of Amsterdam* (Luxembourg: European Commission, Office for Official Publications of the European Community).

Evaluation Partnership (2010) *Evaluation of the European Platform for Action on Diet, Physical Activity and Health* (Brussels: European Commission).

Evans, D. (2003) 'Taking public health out of the ghetto: the policy and practice of multidisciplinary public health in the UK', *Social Science and Medicine*, 57, 959–67.

Evans, D. and Forbes, T. (2009) 'Partnerships in health and social care: England and Scotland compared', *Public Policy and Administration*, 24(1), 67–83.

Evans, R. (2008) 'Thomas McKeown, meet Fidel Castro: physicians, population health and the Cuban paradox', *Healthcare Policy*, 3(4), 21–32.

Exworthy, M. and Hunter, D. (2012) 'The challenge of joined up government in tackling health inequalities', *International Journal of Public Administration*, 34, 201–12.

Faculty of Public Health (2008) *Specialist Public Health Workforce in the UK* (London: FPH).

Feingold, E. (1977) 'Citizen participation: a review of the issues'. In Metsch, J., Rosen, H. and Levey, S. (eds) *The Consumer and the Healthcare System: Social and Managerial Perspectives* (New York: Spectrum), pp. 153–60.

Feinsilver, J. (1993) *Healing the Masses: Cuban Health Politics at Home and Abroad* (Berkeley, CA: University of California Press).

Feinsilver, J. (2010) 'Cuba's health politics at home and abroad', *Socialist Register 2010: Morbid Symptoms – Health Under Capitalism*, 46, 216–39.

Felce, D. and Perry, J. (1995) 'Quality of life: its definition and measurement', *Research and Developmental Disabilities*, 16(1), 51–74.

Fenwick, J., Miller, K. and McTavish, D. (2012) 'Co-governance or meta-bureaucracy? Perspectives of local governance partnership in England and Scotland', *Policy and Politics*, 40(3), 405–22.

Finer, S. (1952) *The Life and Times of Sir Edwin Chadwick* (London: Methuen).

Flynn, R., Williams, G. and Pickard, S. (1996) *Markets and Networks: Contracting in Community Health Services* (Buckingham: Open University).

Foley, P. and Martin, S. (2000) 'A new deal for the community? Public participation in regeneration and local service delivery', *Policy and Politics*, 28(4), 479–91.

Fooks, G. (2011) 'Corporate social responsibility and access to policy elites: an analysis of tobacco industry documents', *PLoS Medicine*, 8(8); e1001076 (accessed 22 March 2012).

Fotaki, M. (2007) 'Can directors of public health implement the new public health agenda in primary care?', *Policy and Politics*, 35(2), 311–35.

Freudenberg, N. (2012) 'The manufacture of lifestyle: the role of corporations in unhealthy living', *Journal of Public Health Policy*, 33(2), 244–56.

Friedli, L. (2009) *Mental Health, Resilience and Inequalities* (Copenhagen: WHO Regional Office for Europe).

Friedman, M. (1970) 'The social responsibility of business is to increase its profits', *New York Times Magazine*, 13 September 1970, pp. 32–3.

Frye, M. and Webb, A. (2002) *Working Together: Effective Partnership Working on the Ground* (London: HM Treasury).

Fung, A. (2006) 'Varieties of participation in complex governance', *Public Administration Review*, 66(S1), 66–75.

Funnell, R., Oldfield, K. and Speller, K. (1995) *Towards Healthier Alliances: A Tool for Planning, Evaluating and Developing Healthy Alliances* (London: Health Education Authority).

Gerrard, M. (2006) *A Stifled Voice: CHC in England 1974–2003* (Brighton: Pen Press).

Giddens, A. (1999) *Runaway World: How Globalization Is Reshaping Our Lives* (London: Profile).

Gidley, B. (2007) 'Sure Start: an upstream approach to reducing health inequalities?' In Scriven, A. and Garman, S. (eds) *Public Health: Social Context and Action* (Maidenhead: Open University Press), pp. 144–53.

Gilchrist, A. (2003) 'Community development and networking for health'. In Orme, J., Powell, J., Harrison, T. and Grey, M. (eds) *Public Health for the 21st Century: New Perspectives on Policy, Participation and Practice* (Maidenhead: Open University Press), pp. 145–59.

Gilchrist, A. (2006) 'Partnership and participation: power in process', *Public Policy and Administration*, 21(3), 71–85.

Gilmore, A. and Fooks, G. (2012) 'Global Fund needs to address conflict of interest', *Bulletin of the World Health Organization*, 90, 71–2.

Glasby, J. and Dickinson, H. (2008) *Partnership Working in Health and Social Care* (Bristol: Policy Press).

Glasby, J. and Peck, E. (2003) *Care Trusts: Partnership Working in Action* (Abingdon: Radcliffe Medical Press).

Glendinning, C., Powell, M. and Rummery, K. (eds) (2002) *Partnerships, New Labour and the Governance of Welfare* (Bristol: Policy Press).

Gostin, L., Ooms, G., Heywood, M., Haffeld, J., Mogedal, S., Rottingen, J-A. et al. (2010) *The Joint Action and Learning Initiative on National and Global Responsibilities for Health*. Background Paper No. 53 (Geneva: WHO).

Grabosky, P. and Braithwaite, J. (1986) *Of Manners Gentle: Enforcement Strategies of Australian Business Regulatory Agencies* (Melbourne: Oxford University Press).

Gray, B. (1989) *Collaborating: Finding Common Ground for Multiparty Problems* (San Francisco: Jossey Bass).

Green, C. and Drakeford, M. (2001) 'Wales: Assemblies and action'. In Centre for Civil Society and NCVO, *Next Steps in Voluntary Action* (London: NCVO), pp. 97–116.

Greene, R. (2003) 'Effective community health participation strategies: a Cuban example', *International Journal of Health Planning and Management*, 18(2), 105–16.

Greer, S. (2009a) *The Politics of European Union Health Policies* (Buckingham: Open University Press).

Greer, S. (2009b) *Territorial Politics and Health Policy* (Manchester: Manchester University Press).

Greer, S., Donnelly, P., Wilson, I. and Stewart, E. (2011) *Health Board Elections and Alternative Pilots in NHS Scotland: An Interim Report* (Edinburgh: Scottish Government).

Griffiths, J. and Dark, P. (2006) *Shaping the Future of Public Health: Promoting Health in the NHS* (London: DH).

Gustafson, U. and Driver, S. (2005) 'Parents, power and public participation: Sure Start, an experiment in New Labour governance', *Social Policy and Administration*, 39(5), 528–43.

Ham, C. and Ellins, J. (2010) 'Employee ownership in the NHS', *BMJ*, 341, 1176.

Hancock, T. (1998) 'Caveat partner: reflections on partnership with the private sector', *Health Promotion International*, 13(3), 193–5.

Handsley, S. (2007) 'Community involvement and civil engagement in multidisciplinary public health'. In Lloyd, C., Handsley, S., Douglas, J., Earle, S. and Spurr, S. (eds) *Policy and Practice in Promoting Public Health* (London: Sage/Open University), pp. 223–56.

Hanratty, B., Milton, B., Ashton, M. and Whitehead, M. (2012) 'McDonalds and KFC, it's never going to happen: the challenges of working with food outlets to tackle the obesogenic environment', *Journal of Public Health*, 34(4), 548–54.

Harding, E. and Kane, M. (2011) 'Joint strategic needs assessment: reconciling new expectation with reality', *Journal of Integrated Care*, 19(6), 37–44.

Hardy, B., Hudson, B. and Warrington, C. (2000) *The Nuffield Partnership Assessment Tool* (Leeds: Nuffield Institute for Health).

Harkins, C. (2010) 'The Portman Group', *BMJ*, 340, b5659, 20 January (accessed 23 August 2011).

Harris, B. (2010) 'Voluntary action and the state in historical perspective', *Voluntary Sector Review*, 1(1), 25–40.

Harris, E., Wise, M., Hawe, P., Finlay, P. and Nutbeam, D. (1995) *Working Together: Intersectoral Action for Health* (Canberra: Australian Government Publishing Service).

Hastings, G. (2012) 'Why corporate power is a public health priority', *BMJ*, 345 e5124, 21 August (accessed 22 February 2013).

Hawkins, B., Holden, C. and McCambridge, J. (2012) 'Alcohol industry influence on UK alcohol policy: a new research agenda for public health', *Critical Public Health*, 22(3), 297–305.

Haynes, P. (2009) *Before Going Further with Social Capital – Eight Key Criteria to Address* (University of Valencia: INGENIO).

Healthcare Commission (2009) *Listening, Learning, Working Together* (London: Healthcare Commission).

Healthcare Commission and Audit Commission (2008) *Are We Choosing Health? The Impact of Policy on the Delivery of Health Improvement Programmes and Services* (London: Commission for Healthcare Audit and Inspection).

Health Committee (2001) *Public Health. 2nd Report 2000-1*. HC 30 (London: TSO).

Health Committee (2003) *Patient and Public Involvement in the NHS. 7th Report 2002–3*. HC 697 (London: TSO).

Health Committee (2007) *Patient and Public Involvement in the NHS. 3rd Report 2006–7*. HC 278 (London: TSO).

Health Committee (2009) *Health Inequalities. 3rd Report 2008–9*. HC 286 (London: TSO).

Health Committee (2010) *Alcohol. 1st Report 2009–10.* HC 151 (London:TSO).

Health Committee (2011a) *Public Health. 12th Report 2010–11.* HC 1048 (London:TSO).

Health Committee (2011b) *Commissioning: Further Issues. 5th Report 2010–11.* HC 796 (London: TSO).

Health Committee (2012a) *Social Care. 14th Report 2010–12.* HC1583 (London:TSO).

Health Committee (2012b) *Government's Alcohol Strategy. 3rd Report 2012–13.* HC 132 (London: TSO).

Health Targets and Implementation Committee (1988) *Health for Australians* (Canberra: Australian Government Printing Service).

Hearn, S., Martin, H, Signal, L. and Wise, M. (2005) 'Health promotion in Australia and New Zealand: the struggle for equity'. In Scriven, E. and Garman, S. (eds) *Promoting Health: Global Perspectives* (Palgrave: Basingstoke), pp. 239–48.

Heenan, D. and Birrell, D. (2006) 'The integration of health and social care: the lessons from Northern Ireland', *Social Policy and Administration*, 40(1), 47–66.

Held, D. and McGrew, A. (2000) *The Global Transformations Reader* (London: Polity Press).

Heritage, Z. and Dooris, M. (2009) 'Community participation and empowerment in healthy cities', *Health Promotion International*, 24 S1, pi45–55 (doi:10.1093/heapro/dap054; accessed 20 February 2012).

Hills, D., Elliott, E., Kowarzic, U., Sullivan, F., Stern, E., Platt S. et al. (2007) 'The evaluation of the Big Lottery Fund Healthy Living Centres Programme (Bridge Consortium)' (www. biglotteryfund.org.uk/hi/er_eval_hlc_final_report.pdf9; accessed 25 January 2012).

Hilton, M. and McKay, J. (eds) (2011) *The Ages of Voluntarism* (Oxford: Oxford University Press).

HM Government (2005) *Health, Work and Well-Being: Caring for our Future. A Strategy for the Heath and Well-Being of Working Age People* (London:TSO).

HM Government (2007a) *PSA Delivery Agreement 21: Build More Cohesive, Empowered and Active Communities* (London: HM Treasury).

HM Government (2007b) *Safe. Sensible. Social. Next Steps in the National Alcohol Strategy* (London: DH).

HM Government (2008a) *Healthy Weight, Healthy Lives* (London: HM Government).

HM Government (2008b) *Health is Global: A UK Government Strategy 2008–13* (London:TSO).

HM Government (2010a) *The Coalition: Our Programme for Government* (London: Cabinet Office).

HM Government (2010b) *The Compact* (London: Cabinet Office).

HM Treasury (2002) *The Role of the Voluntary and Community Sector in Service Delivery: A Cross-cutting Review* (London: HM Treasury).

Hodgkinson, R. (1967) *The Origins of the NHS: The Medical Services of the New Poor Law* (London: Wellcome Foundation).

Hodgson, L. (2004) 'Manufactured civil society: counting the cost', *Critical Social Policy*, 24(2), 139–64.

Hogg, C. (2009) *Citizens, Consumers and the NHS: Capturing Voices* (Basingstoke: Palgrave).

Hogg, E. and Baines, S. (2011) 'Changing responsibilities and roles of the voluntary and community sector in the welfare mix: a review', *Social Policy and Society*, 10(3), 341–52.

Hogstedt, C., Moberg, H., Lundgren, B. and Backhans, M. (2008) *Health for All? A Critical Analysis of Public Health Policies in Eight European Countries* (Ostersund: Swedish National Institute for Public Health).

Hollis, P. (1974) *Pressure from Without in Early Victorian England* (London: Edward Arnold).

Home Office (1990) *Efficiency Scrutiny of Government Funding of the Voluntary Sector* (London: Home Office).

Home Office (2004) *Change Up: Capacity Building and Infrastructure Framework for the Voluntary and Community Sector* (London: Home Office).

Horrigan, B. (2010) *Corporate Social Responsibility in the 21st Century* (Brighton: Edward Elgar).

House of Lords Select Committee on Science and Technology (2011) *Behaviour Change. 2nd Report 2010–12.* HL 179 (London: TSO).

Hudson, B. (1987) 'Collaboration in social welfare: a framework for analysis', *Policy and Politics*, 15(3), 175–82.

Hudson, B. (1995) 'Joint commissioning: organisational revolution or misplaced enthusiasm', *Policy and Politics*, 23(3), 233–49.

Hudson, B. (2011) 'Big Society: a concept in pursuit of a definition', *Journal of Integrated Care*, 19(5), 17–24.

Hudson, B. and Hardy, B. (2002) 'What is a successful partnership and how can it be measured?' In Glendinning, C., Powell, M. and Rummery, K. (eds) *Partnerships, New Labour and Governance* (Bristol: Policy Press), pp. 51–66.

Hudson, B., Hardy, B., Henwood, M. and Wistow, G. (1997) 'Working across professional boundaries: primary health care and social care', *Public Money and Management*, 17(4), 25–30.

Hughes, D. (2009) *Joint Strategic Needs Assessment: Progress So Far* (London: Improvement and Development Agency).

Hughes, D., Mullen, C. and Vincent-Jones, P. (2009) 'Choice v voice: PPI policies and the repositioning of the state in England and Wales', *Health Expectations*, 12, 237–50.

Humphries, R., Galea, A, Sonola, L. and Mundle, C. (2012) *Health and Wellbeing Boards: Systems Leaders or Talking Shops?* (London: King's Fund).

Hunter, D., Marks, L and Smith, K. (2007) *The Public Health System in England: A Scoping Study: Part 2* (Durham: Centre for Public Policy in Health, Durham University).

Hunter, D., Marks, L. and Smith, K. (2010) *The Public Health System in England* (Bristol: Policy Press).

Hunter, D., Perkins, N., Bambra, C., Marks, L., Hopkins, T. and Blackman, T. (2011) *Partnership Working and the Implications for Governance: Issues Affecting Public Health Partnerships* (Southampton: NIHR Service Delivery and Organisation Programme/HMSO).

Huppert, F., Baylis, N. and Keverne, B. (2005) *The Science of Wellbeing* (Oxford: Oxford University Press).

Huxham, C. (2003) 'Theorising collaboration in practice', *Public Management Review*, 5(3), 401–23.

IDeA (Improvement and Development Agency) (2010) *A Glass Half Full: How an Asset Approach Can Improve Community Health and Wellbeing* (London: IDeA).

IDeA (2012) 'Private sector health initiatives' (www.idea.gov.uk; accessed 2 April 2012).

IFF Research (2007) *Third Sector Mapping Research* (London: DH).

Independence Panel (2012) *Protecting Independence: the Voluntary Sector in 2012* (London: Baring Foundation).

Institute of Medicine (1988) *The Future of Public Health* (Washington, DC: National Academies Press).

Institute of Medicine (2002) *The Future of the Public's Health in the 21st Century* (Washington, DC: National Academies Press).

Institute for Public Policy Research, Commission on Public–Private Partnerships (2001) *Building Better Partnerships* (London: Institute for Public Policy Research).

International Health Impact Assessment Consortium (2004) *European Policy Health Impact Assessment: A Guide* (Brussels: European Commission).

Ipsos MORI (2011) *National Survey of Charities and Social Enterprises 2010* (London: Ipsos MORI/Cabinet Office).

Irvine, R. and Stansbury, J. (2004) 'Citizen participation in decision making: is it worth the effort?', *Public Administration Review*, 64(1), 55–64.

Jackson, M. (2010) 'Matching rhetoric with reality: the challenge for Third Sector involvement in local governance', *International Journal of Sociology and Social Policy*, 30(1/2), 17–31.

Jacques, H. (2013) 'Government considers statutory regulation of public health professionals', *BMJ Careers*, 14 January (http://careers.bmj.com; accessed 22 May 2013).

Jebb, S., Ahern, A.L., Olson, A.D., Aston, L.M., Holzapfel, C., Stoll, J. et al. (2011) 'Primary care referral to a commercial provider for weight loss: treatment versus standard care: a randomised controlled trial', *Lancet*, 378, 1485–92.

Jewkes, R. and Murcott, A. (1998) 'Community representatives: representing the community?', *Social Science and Medicine*, 46(7), 843–58.

Johnson, C., Coleman, A., Boyd, A., Bradshaw, D., Gains, F., Shacklady-Smith, A. et al. (2007) *Scrutinising for Health* (Manchester: University of Manchester).

Johnston, G. and Percy-Smith, J. (2003) 'In search of social capital', *Policy and Politics*, 31(3), 321–34.

Jones, G. and Stewart, J. (2009) 'New development: accountability in public partnerships – the case of local strategic partnerships', *Public Money and Management*, 29(1), 59–64.

Jones, J. and Barry, M. (2011) 'Developing a scale to measure trust in health promotion partnerships', *Health Promotion International*, 26(4), 484–91.

Judge, K. and Bauld, L. (2007) 'Learning from policy failure? Health action zones in England', *European Journal of Public Health*, 16(4), 341–4.

Kahneman, D., Diener, E. and Schwartz, N. (eds) (2003) *Wellbeing: The Foundations of Hedonic Psychology* (New York: Russell Sage).

Kane, J., Clarke, J., Lesniewski, S., Wilton, J., Pratten, B., and Wilding, K. (2009) *The UK Civil Society Almanac 2009* (London: NVCO).

Kane, D. and Allen, J. (2011) *Counting the Cuts: The Impact of Spending Cuts on the UK Voluntary and Community Sector* (London: NCVO).

Kane, P. (2008) 'Sure Start Local Programmes in England', *Lancet*, 372, 1610–11.

Kaplan, G.A., Pamuk, E.R., Lynch, J.W., Cohen, R.D. and Balfour, J.L. (1996) 'Inequality in income and mortality in the United States: analysis of mortality and potential pathways', *BMJ*, 312, 999–1003.

Kath, E. (2011) 'Revolutionary health: state capacity, popular participation, the Cuban paradox', *Journal of Iberian and Latin American Research*, 17(2), 213–29.

Kaul, I. Grunberg, I. and Stern, M. (eds) (1999) *Global Public Goods: International Cooperation in the 21st Century* (UN Development Programme).

Kawachi, I. and Berkman, L. (eds) (2003) *Neighbourhoods and Health* (Oxford: Oxford University Press).

Kearney, J. and Williamson, A. (2001) 'Northern Ireland: the delayed devolution'. In Centre for Civil Society and NCVO, *Next Steps in Voluntary Action* (London: NCVO), pp. 57–70.

Kelly, J. (2007) 'Reforming public services in the UK: bringing in the Third Sector', *Public Administration*, 85(4), 1003–22.

Kendall, J. (2009) 'The third sector and the policy process in the UK: ingredients in a hyperactive horizontal policy environment'. In Kendall, J. (ed.) *Handbook of Third Sector Policy in Europe* (Cheltenham: Edward Elgar).

Kendall, J. and Knapp, M. (1995) 'A loose and baggy monster'. In Davis Smith, J., Rochester, C. and Hedley, R. (eds) *An Introduction to the Voluntary Sector* (London: Routledge), pp. 66–95.

Kennedy, H. (2007) *Report of the Advisory Group on Campaigning and the Voluntary Sector* (chair Baroness Kennedy) (www.ncvo-vol.org.uk/sites/default/files/Advisory_Group_on_Campaigning_Report_2007.pdf; accessed 30 May 2012).

Kerr, D. (2005) *A Report on the Future of the NHS in Scotland: Building a Health Service Fit for the Future* (Edinburgh: Scottish Executive).

Kickbusch, I. and de Leeuw, E. (1999) 'Global public health: revisiting healthy public policy at the global level', *Health Promotion International*, 14(4), 285–8.

Kickbusch, I. and Payne, L. (2004) 'Constructing global public health in the 21st century'. In *Meeting on Global Health Governance and Accountability*, 2–3 June 2004 (Cambridge, MA: Harvard University).

Kickbusch, I. and Seck, B. (2007) 'Global public health'. In Douglas, J., Earle, S., Handlsey, S., Lloyd, C., and Spurr, S. (2007) *A Reader in Promoting Public Health: Challenge and Controversy* (London: Sage/Open University), pp. 159–68.

Kirk, J. and Erisman, M. (2009) *Cuban Medical Internationalism: Origins, Evolution and Goals* (New York: Palgrave Macmillan).

Klawiter, M. (1999) 'Racing for the cure, walking women and toxic touring: mapping cultures of action within the Bay Area terrain of breast cancer', *Social Problems*, 46(1), 104–26.

Klein, R. (1983) *The Politics of the National Health Service* (London: Longman).

Knight, B. (1993) *Voluntary Action* (London: Centris).

Koivusalo, M. (2006) 'The impact of economic globalisation on health', *Theoretical Medicine and Bioethics*, 27, 1–34.

Kooiman, J. (2003) *Governing as Governance* (London: Sage).

Kreuter, M., Lezin, N. and Young, L. (2000) 'Evaluating community based collaborative mechanisms: implications for practitioners', *Health Promotion Practice*, 1(1), 49–63.

Kuznetsova, D. (2012) *Healthy Places: Councils Leading on Public Health* (London: New Local Government Network).

Labonte, R. and Schrecker, T. (2004) 'Committed to health for all?: How the G7/G8 rate', *Social Science and Medicine*, 59, 1661–76.

Labour Party (1997) *Building the Future Together* (London: Labour Party).

Lalonde, M. (1974) *A New Perspective on the Health of Canadians* (Ottawa: Ministry of National Health and Welfare).

Lancet (2011) 'Two days in New York: reflection on the UN NCD summit,' *Lancet Oncology*, 12(11), 981.

Lancet (2012) 'The breast cancer screening debate: closing a chapter?', *Lancet*, 380, 1714.

Lancet/UCL Institute for Global Health Commission (2009) 'Managing the health effects of climate change', *Lancet*, 373, 1693–73.

Lang, T. and Heasman, M. (2004) *Food Wars: The Global Battle for Mouths, Minds, and Markets* (London: Earthscan).

Lang, T. and Rayner, G. (2012) 'Ecological public health: the 21st century's big idea?', *BMJ*, 345, e5466, 21 August (accessed 5 June, 2013).

Lang, T., Barling, D. and Caraher, M. (2009) *Food Policy: Integrating Health, Society and the Environment* (Oxford: Oxford University Press).

Langmore, J. and Fitzgerald, S. (2010) 'Global economic governance: addressing the democratic deficit', *Development*, 53(3), 390–3.

Lansley, A. (2011) 'The role of business in public health', *Lancet*, 377, 121.

Lasker, R., Weiss, E. and Miller, R. (2001) 'Partnership synergy: a practical framework for studying and strengthening the collaborative advantage', *Milbank Quarterly*, 79, 179–205.

Laverack, C. (2005) *Power, Empowerment and Professional Practice* (London: Palgrave).

Layne, L. (2006) Pregnancy and infant loss support: a new, feminist, American patient movement?', *Social Science and Medicine*, 62, 602–13.

Lear, J. and Mossialos, E. (2008) 'EU Law and health policy in Europe', *Euro Observer*, 10(3), 1–3.

Learmonth, M., Martin, G. and Warwick, P. (2009) 'Ordinary and effective: the Catch-22 in managing the public voice in health care?', *Health Expectations*, 12(1), 106–15.

Lee, K. (2009) *The World Health Organization* (London: Routledge).

Lee, K. and Collin, J. (eds) (2005) *Global Change and Health* (Maidenhead: Open University Press).

Lee, K., Sridhar, D. and Patel, M. (2009) 'Bridging the divide: global governance of trade and health', *Lancet*, 373, 416–22.

Legge, D. (2012) 'The future of WHO hangs in the balance', *BMJ*, 345, e6877, 25 October (accessed 24 January 2012).

Lewis, J. (1986) *What Price Community Medicine?* (Brighton: Wheatsheaf).

Lewis, J. (1999) 'Reviewing the relationship between the voluntary sector and the state in Britain in the 1990s', *Voluntas*, 10(3), 255–70.

Lewis, J. (2005) 'New Labour's approach to the voluntary sector: independence and the meaning of partnership', *Social Policy and Society*, 4(2), 121–33.

Lewis, R., Hunt, P. and Carson, D. (2006) *Social Enterprise and Community Based Care* (London: King's Fund).

LGA (Local Government Association) (2008) *Report of the Local Government Commission on Health* (London: LGA).

LGA (2011a) *Communities for Health: How Health and Wellbeing Became Everyone's Business* (London: LGA).

LGA (2011b) *Communities for Health: Final Evaluation* (London: LGA).

LGA/DH (2012) *Resource Sheet 6: Collaboration Through Public Health Networks* (London: LGA).

LGA/Centre for Public Scrutiny (2012) *Local Healthwatch, Health and Wellbeing Boards and Health Scrutiny* (London: LGA).

LGA/Regional Voices/NHS Institute for Innovation and Improvement (2012a) *Building Successful Healthwatch Organisations* (London: LGA).

LGA/Regional Voices/NHS Institute for Innovation and Improvement (2012b) *Supporting Healthwatch Pathfinders: Healthwatch Pathfinder National Learning Network Final Report* (London: LGA).

LGA/UK Public Health Alliance/NHS Confederation (2004) *Releasing the Potential for the Public's Health* (London: LGA/UKPHA/NHS Confederation).

Li, Y. (2007) 'Social capital, social exclusion and wellbeing'. In Scriven, A. and Garman, S. (eds) *Public Health: Social Context and Action* (Maidenhead: Open University Press), pp. 60–75.

Liberal Democrats (2008) *Empowerment, Fairness and Quality in Healthcare* (London: Liberal Democrats).

Liberal Democrats (2010) *Manifesto 2010* (London: Liberal Democrats).

Lightsey, D., McQueen, D. and Anderson, L. (2005) 'Health promotion in the USA: building a science-based health promotion policy'. In Scriven, A. and Garman, S. (eds) *Promoting Health: Global Perspectives* (Palgrave: Basingstoke), pp. 266–78.

Limb, M. (2012) 'Health campaigners attack government plans to remove calories from food as "token gestures"', *BMJ*, 344, e2332 (accessed 18 April 2012).

Lin, V. (2007) 'Health promotion in Australia: twenty years on from the Ottawa charter', *Promotion and Education*, XIV(4), 203–8.

Ling, T. (2000) 'Unpacking partnership: the case of health care'. In Clarke, J., Gewirtz, S. and McLaughlin E. (eds) *New Managerialism, New Welfare* (London: Sage), pp. 82–101.

Litva, A., Canvin, K., Shepherd, M., Jacoby, A. and Gabbay, M. (2009) 'Lay perceptions of the desired role and type of user involvement in clinical governance', *Health Expectations*, 12(1), 81–91.

Local Government Information Unit (2010) *All's Well That End's Well?: Local Government Leading on Health Improvement* (London: LGIU).

Lock, S. and McKee, M. (2005) 'Health impact assessment: assessing opportunities and barriers to intersectoral health improvement in an expanded European Union', *Journal of Epidemiology and Public Health*, 59, 356–360.

Loewenstein, G., Asche, D., Friedman, J., Melichar, L. and Volpp. K. (2012) 'Can behavioural economics make us healthier?', *BMJ*, 344, e3482, 23 May (accessed 21 February 2013).

Long, S. (1999) 'The tyranny of the customer and the cost of consumerism: an analysis using systems and psychoanalytic approaches to groups and society', *Human Relations*, 52(6), 723–43.

Longmate, N. (1966) *King Cholera: The Biography of a Disease* (London: Hamish Hamilton).

Lord Laming (2009) *The Protection of Children in England: A Progress Report*. HC 330 (London: TSO).

Loughborough University (2008) *Well@Work Evaluation* (London: British Heart Foundation).

Lowndes, V. and Skelcher, C. (1998) 'The dynamics of multi-organisational partnerships: an analysis of changing modes of governance', *Public Administration*, 76, 313–33.

Lowndes, V., Pratchett, L. and Stoker, G. (2001a) 'Trends in participation: local government perspectives', *Public Administration*, 79(1) 205–22.

Lowndes, V., Pratchett, L. and Stoker, G. (2001b) 'Trends in participation: citizens' perspectives', *Public Administration*, 79(2), 455–5.

Ludlam, S. and Smith, M. (eds) (2004) *Governing as New Labour: Policy and Politics under Blair* (Basingstoke: Palgrave).

Lyon, F. and Sepulveda, L. (2009) 'Mapping social enterprises: past approaches, challenges and future directions', *Social Enterprise Journal*, 5(1), 83–94.

MacDonagh, O. (1977) *Early Victorian Government* (London: Weidenfield & Nicolson).

Macintyre, K. and Hadad, J. (2002) 'Cuba'. In Fried, B. and Gaydos, L. (eds) *World Health Systems: Challenges and Perspectives* (Chicago: Health Administration Press), pp. 445–61.

Mackenzie, M., O'Donnell, C., Halliday, E., Sridharan, S. and Platt, S. (2010) 'Do health improvement programmes fit in with MRC guidance on evaluating complex interventions?', *BMJ*, 340, c185, 1 February (accessed 28 February 2013).

Mackereth, C. (2006) *Community Development: New Challenges, New Opportunities* (London: Community Practitioners' and Health Visitors' Association).

Mackey, T. and Liang, B. (2013) 'A United Nations global health panel for global health governance', *Social Science and Medicine*, 76, 12–15.

Macmillan, R. (2010) *The Third Sector Delivering Public Services: An Evidence Review* (Birmingham: Third Sector Research Centre).

Mallinson, S., Popay, J., Kowarzik, U. and Mackian, S. (2006) 'Developing the public health workforce: a communities of practice perspective', *Policy and Politics*, 34(2), 265–85.

Manokha, I. (2004) 'Corporate social responsibility: a new signifier? An analysis of business ethics and good business practice', *Politics*, 24(1), 56–64.

Marks, L. (2007) 'Fault lines between policy and practice in local partnerships', *Journal of Health Organisation and Management*, 21(2), 136–48.

Marks, L. and Hunter, D. (2007) *Social Enterprises and the NHS: Changing Patterns of Ownership and Accountability* (London: Unison).

Marks, L., Cave, S., Hunter, D., Mason, J. and Peckham, S. (2011) 'Governance for health and wellbeing in the English NHS', *Journal of Health Services Research and Policy*, 16, 14–21.

Marshall, K. (2008) *The World Bank* (London: Routledge).

Martikke, S. and Moxham, C. (2010) 'Public sector commissioning: experiences of voluntary organisations delivering health and social services', *International Journal of Public Administration*, 33(14), 790–9.

Martin, G. (2008) 'Ordinary people only; knowledge, representativeness and the publics of patient participation in health care', *Sociology of Health and Illness*, 30(1), 35–54.

Maryon-Davis, A. (2011) 'We could be creating a monster', *Health Service Journal*, 3 February, 14.

Matka, E., Barnes, M. and Sullivan, H. (2002) 'Health action zones: creating alliances to achieve change', *Policy Studies*, 23, 97–106.

Mattesich, P., Murray-Close, M. and Monsey, B. (2001) *Collaboration – What Makes it Work?* (2nd edn) (St Paul, MN: Wilder Foundation).

Mayor, S. (2004) 'Researcher objects to drink industry representative sitting on alcohol research body', *BMJ*, 329, 71.

McCarthy, M. (2007) 'The Global Fund 5 years on', *Lancet*, 370, 307–8.

McCulloch, A. (2001) 'Social environments and health: cross sectional national survey', *BMJ*, 323, 208–9.

McGarrity, T. and Wagner, W. (2008) *Bending Science: How Special Interests Corrupt Public Health Research* (Cambridge, MA: Harvard University Press).

McKee, M. (2007) 'International Public Health'. In Hunter, D. and Griffiths, S. (eds) *New Perspectives in Public Health* (2nd edn) (Oxford: Radcliffe Medical Press), pp. 71–6.

McKee, M., Hurst, L., Aldridge, R., Raine, R., Mindell, J., Wolfe, I. et al. (2011) 'Public health in England: an option for the way forward?', *Lancet*, 378, 536–49.

McKinsey and Co. (2002) *Developing Successful Global Health Alliances* (Seattle: Bill and Melinda Gates Foundation).

McMurray, R. (2007) 'Our reforms, our partnerships, same problems: the chronic case of the English NHS', *Public Money and Management*, February, 77–82.

Melhuish, E., Belsky, J., Leyland, A. and Barnes, J. (2008) 'Effects of fully-established Sure Start local programmes on 3 year old children and their families living in England: a quasi-experimental observational study', *Lancet*, 372, 1641–7.

Mid Staffordshire Foundation Trust Public Inquiry (2013) *Report: Executive Summary*. HC 947 (London: TSO).

Milio, N. (1986) *Promoting Health Through Public Policy* (Ottawa: Canadian Public Health Association).

Miller, C. and Ahmad, Y. (2000) 'Collaboration and partnership: an effective response to complexity and fragmentation or solution built on sand?', *International Journal on Sociology and Social Policy*, 20(5–6), 1–38.

Miller, D. and Harkins, C. (2010) 'Corporate strategy, corporate capture: food and alcohol industry lobbying and public health', *Critical Social Policy*, 30(4), 564–89.

Miller, P. and Rose, N. (2008) *Governing the Present* (Oxford: Polity Press).

Mills, M. (1992) *The Politics of Dietary Change* (Aldershot: Dartmouth).

Minister of Health (Canada) (2005) *The Integrated Pan Canadian Healthy Living Strategy* (www.phac-aspc.gc.ca/hl-vs-strat/pdf/hls_e.pdf; accessed 16 December 2010).

Ministers of Foreign Affairs Norway, France, Thailand, South Africa, Brazil, Indonesia, and Senegal (2007) 'Oslo Ministerial Declaration – global health: a pressing foreign policy issue of our time', *Lancet*, 368, 373–8.

Ministry of Health Services, British Columbia (2005) *A Framework for Core Functions in Public Health: Resource Document* (British Columbia: Ministry of Health Service).

Ministry of Social Affairs and Health (2001) *Health 2015 Public Health Programme* (Helsinki: Finnish Ministry of Social Affairs and Health).

Mitchell, A. and Voon, T. (2011) 'Implications of the World Trade Organization in combating non-communicable diseases', *Public Health*, 125, 832–9.

Mold, A. and Berridge, V. (2008) 'The rise of the user? Voluntary organisations, the state and illegal drugs in England since the 1960s', *Drugs: Education, Prevention and Policy*, 15(5), 451–61.

Moon, G. and North, N. (2000) *Policy and Place: General Medical Practice in the UK* (Basingstoke: Palgrave).

Moran, M. (2003) *The British Regulatory State* (Oxford: Oxford University Press).

Morgan, A. and Popay, J. (2007) 'Community participation for health: reducing health inequalities and building social capital'. In Scriven, A. and Garman, S. (eds) *Public Health: Social Context and Action* (Maidenhead: Open University Press), pp. 154–65.

Morison, J. (2000) 'The government–voluntary sector compacts: governance, governmentality, and civil society', *Journal of Law and Society*, 27(1), 98–132.

Moss-Kanter, R. (1994) 'Collaborative advantage: the art of alliances', *Harvard Business Review*, 72(4), 96–108.

Muntaner, C., Lynch, J. and Davey Smith, G. (2001) 'Social capital, disorganised communities, and the Third Way', *International Journal of Health Services*, 31(2), 213–37.

Myers, P., Barnes, J. and Brodie, I. (2004) *Partnership Working in Sure Start Programmes: Early Findings from Local Programme Evaluations* (London: Institute of Children, Families and Social Issues).

Naidoo, J. and Wills, J. (2005) *Public Health and Health Promotion; Developing Practice* (2nd edn) (London: Baillière Tindall).

Naidoo, J., Orme , J. and Barrett, G. (2003) 'Capacity and capability in public health'. In Orme, J., Powell, J., Taylor, P., Harrison, T. and Grey, M. (eds) *Public Health for the 21st Century* (Berkshire: Open University Press), pp. 79–92.

NAO (National Audit Office) (2005) *Working with the Third Sector. Session 2005–6.* HC 75 (London: TSO).

NAO (2007) *Local Area Agreements and Third Sector Public Service Delivery* (London: TSO).

NAO (2009) *Building the Capacity of the Third Sector.* HC 132 2008–9 (London: TSO).

NAO (2012) *Central Government's Implementation of the National Compact* (London: NAO).

National Advisory Committee on SARS and Public Health (2003) *Learning from SARS – Renewal of Public Health in Canada* (chair D. Naylor) (Ottawa: Health Canada).

National Assembly for Wales (2001) *Improving Health in Wales* (Cardiff: National Assembly for Wales).

National Assembly for Wales/Office for Public Management (2002) *Signposts: A Practical Guide to Patient and Public Involvement in Wales* (London/Cardiff: OPM/NAfW).

National Screening Committee (2010) *Advice on Private Screening Being Offered Through GP Practices* (www.screening.nhs.uk/private-screening; accessed 10 May 2010).

NAVCA (National Association for Voluntary and Community Action) (2011) *NAVCA Members and Representation* (Sheffield: NAVCA).

NCC (National Consumer Council) (2005) *Three Steps to Credible Self Regulation* (London: NCC).

NCC/Involve (2008) *Deliberative Public Engagement* (London: NCC).

Needham, C. (2002) 'Consultation: a cure for local government', *Parliamentary Affairs*, 55(4), 699–714.

NEF (New Economics Foundation) (2010) *Cutting It* (London: NEF).

Nettleton, S. and Burrows, R. (1997) 'Knit your own without a pattern: health promotion specialists in an internal market', *Social Policy and Administration*, 31(2), 191–201.

Newman, J. (2001) *Modernising Governance: New Labour, Policy and Society* (London: Sage).

Newman, J. and Clarke, J. (2009) *Publics, Politics and Power: Remaking the Public in Public Services* (London: Sage).

NHS Confederation/Department of Health/Local Government Improvement and Development/SOLACE/Royal Society for Public Health/Association of Directors of Childrens Services/Association of Directors of Public Health/NHS Alliance/Royal College of General Practitioners (2011) *Operating Principles for Health and Wellbeing Boards* (London: NHS Confederation).

NHS Confederation/Department of Health/SOLACE/Royal Society for Public Health/ Association of Directors of Public Health/NHS Alliance/NHS Clinical Commissioners/ National Association of Primary Care/Regional Voices/Faculty of Public Health/NHS Institute for Innovation and Improvement/Association of Directors of Adult Social Services/ Local Government Association (2012a) *Operating Principles for Joint Strategic Needs Assessments and Joint Health and Wellbeing Strategies* (London: NHS Confederation).

NHS Confederation/Department of Health/Local Government Association/NHS Institute for Innovation and Improvement (2012b) *Support and Resources for Health and Wellbeing Boards* (London: NHS Confederation).

NHS Confederation/Department of Health/Local Government Association/NHS Institute for Innovation and Improvement (2012c) *Improving Population Health: Action Learning for Health and Wellbeing Boards* (London: NHS Confederation).

NHS Confederation/Department of Health/Local Government Association/NHS Institute for Innovation and Improvement (2012d) *Encouraging Integrated Working to Improve Services for Adults and Older People* (London: NHS Confederation).

NHS Executive (1996) *Patient Partnership: Building a Collaborative Strategy* (Leeds: DH).

NHS Executive/Institute of Health Service Management/NHS Confederation (1998) *In the Public Interest: Developing a Strategy for Patient Partnership in the NHS* (Leeds: NHS Executive).

NHS Future Forum (2011a) *Summary Report on Proposed Changes to the NHS* (London: DH).

NHS Future Forum (2011b) *Patient Involvement and Public Accountability* (London: DH).

NHS Future Forum (2012) *The NHS's Role in Public Health* (London: DH).

NHS National Commissioning Board (2012) *Everyone Counts: Planning for Patients 2013–14* (London: NCB).

NHS Workforce Review Team (2009) *Assessment of Workforce Priorities 2009/10* (www.wrt.nhs. uk; accessed 4 May 2010).

NICE (National Institute for Health and Clinical Excellence) (2008a) *Promoting Physical Activity in the Workplace* (London: NICE).

NICE (2008b) *Smoking Cessation Services in Primary Care, Pharmacies, Local Authorities and Workplaces, Particularly for Manual Working Groups, Pregnant Women and Hard to Reach Communities* (London: NICE).

NICE (2008c) *Community Engagement to Improve Health* (London: NICE).

NICE (2009a) *Managing Long Term Sickness Absences and Incapacity for Work* (London: NICE).

NICE (2009b) *Promoting Mental Wellbeing Through Productive and Healthy Working Conditions: Guidance for Employers* (London: NICE).

Nishtar, S. (2004) 'Public-private partnerships in health – a global call to action', *Health Research Policy and Systems*, 2(5), doi: 10.1186/1478-4505-2-5 (accessed 2 April 12).

NLIAH (National Leadership and Innovation Agency for Healthcare) (2009) *Getting Collaboration to Work in Wales: Lessons from the NHS and Partners* (Llanharan: NLIAH).

Norman, J. (2010) *The Big Society* (Buckingham: University of Buckingham Press).

Northover, Baroness (2012) House of Lords Debates, 28 January 2013, column 1312.

NPCRDC (National Primary Care Research and Development Centre) (2006) *The Implementation of Local Authority Scrutiny of Primary Health Care 2002–2005* (Manchester: NPCRDC).

Nuffield Council on Bioethics (2007) *Public Health: Ethical Issues* (London: Nuffield Council on Bioethics).

Nugent, N. (2010) *The Government and Politics of the European Union* (7th edn) (Basingstoke: Palgrave).

Nutbeam, D. (1994) 'Inter-sectoral action for health: making it work', *Health Promotion International*, 9(3), 143–4.

Nutbeam, D. (1999) 'Achieving population health goals: perspectives on measurement and implementation from Australia', *Canadian Journal of Public Health*, 90(Suppl. 1), S43–46.

Nutbeam, D., Wise, M., Bauman, A. and Leeder, S. (1993) *Goals and Targets for Australia's Health in the Year 2000 and Beyond* (Canberra: Australian Government Printing Service).

Nye, J. (2001) 'Globalisation's democratic deficit – how to make international institutions more accountable', *Foreign Affairs*, 80, 2–6.

ODPM (Office of the Deputy Prime Minister) (2003) *Sustainable Communities: Building for the Future* (London: ODPM).

ODPM (2005) *Process Evaluation of Plan Rationalisation: Formative Evaluation of Community Strategies: Review of Community Strategies – Overview of All and More Detailed Assessment of 50* (London: ODPM).

ODPM (2006) *National Evaluation of Local Strategic Partnerships: Formative Evaluation and Action Research Programme* (London: ODPM).

ODPM/DH (2005) *Creating Healthier Communities: A Resource Pack for Local Partnerships* (London: DH).

Office of the Third Sector (2006) *Partnership in Public Services: An Action Plan for Third Sector Involvement* (London: OTS).

OFSTED (2006) *Healthy Schools, Healthy Children?* (Manchester: OFSTED).

Ogus, A. (1997) 'Self-regulation'. In Bouckaert, B. and de Geest, G. (eds) *Encyclopaedia of Law and Economics* (Vol. 5) (Brighton: Edward Elgar).

Oliver, J. (2011) 'This obesity strategy is a cop out', *Guardian: Comment is Free – Word of Mouth Blog 13.10.11* (www.guardian .co.uk; accessed 15 October 2011).

Ollila, E. (2005) 'Global health priorities: priorities of the wealthy?', *Globalisation and Health*, 1(6), 1–6.

Oneplace (2010) *National Overview Report* (oneplace.direct.gov.uk; accessed 8 May 2010).

Osborne, S. and Flynn, N. (1997) 'Managing the innovative capacity of voluntary and non-profit organisations in the provision of public services', *Public Money and Management*, October–December, 31–9.

Osborne, S., Chew, C. and McLaughlin, K. (2008) 'The innovative capacity of voluntary organizations and the provision of public services: a longitudinal approach', Special issue on Innovation in Public Services, *Public Management Review*, 10(1), 51–70.

Ottewill, R. and Wall, A. (1990) *The Growth and Development of the Community Health Services* (Sunderland: Business Education Publishers).

PAC (Public Accounts Committee) (2010) *Tackling Health Inequalities in Areas with the Worst Health and Deprivation. 3rd Report 2011–12.* HC 470 (London: TSO).

Parker, S., Paun, A., McClory, J. and Blatchford, K. (2010) *Shaping Up: A Whitehall for the Future* (London: Institute for Government).

Pate, J., Fischbacher, M. and Mackinnon, J. (2010) 'Health improvement: countervailing pillars of partnership and profession', *Journal of Health Organisation and Management*, 24(2), 200–17.

PatientView (2009) Local healthcare commissioning; Grassroots involvement?, 18 February 2009 (www.rcn.org.yk/newsevents/press_releases/uk; accessed 22 May 2012).

Patients Association (2011) 'Local Involvement Network Report', *Patient Voice*, November, Part 3, 50.

Pattie, C. and Johnston, R. (2011) 'How big is the Big Society?', *Parliamentary Affairs*, 64(3), 403–24.

Pederson, A., Rootman, I. and O'Neill, M. (2005) 'Health promotion in Canada: back to the past or towards a promising future?' In Scriven, A. and Garman, S. (eds) *Promoting Health: Global Perspectives* (Palgrave: Basingstoke), pp. 255–62.

Performance and Innovation Unit (2000) *Wiring it Up* (London: Cabinet Office).

Perkins, N., Smith, K., Hunter, D., Bambra, C. and Joyce, K. (2010) '"What counts is what works?" New Labour and partnerships in public health', *Policy and Politics*, 38(1), 101–17.

Picker Institute (2009) *Patient and Public Engagement: The Early Impact of World Class Commissioning* (Oxford: Picker Institute).

Pierre, J. and Peters, G. (2000) *Governance, Politics and the State* (Basingstoke: Macmillan).

Pigman, G. (2007) *The World Economic Forum: A Multi-stakeholder Approach to Global Governance* (Oxford: Routledge).

Pinet, G. (2003) 'Global partnerships: a key challenge and opportunity for implementation of international health law', *Medicine and Law*, 22(4), 561–77.

Porter, D. (1999) *Health, Civilisation and the State* (London: Routledge).

Porter, P., Ross, L., Chapman, R., Kohatsu, N. and Fox, P. (2008) *Medicine and Public Health Partnerships: Predictors of Success* (http://scholarship.org/uc/item/2ff6c545; accessed 21 March 2011).

Portes, A. (1998) 'Social capital: its origins and applications in modern sociology', *Annual Review of Sociology*, 24, 1–24.

Powell, M. (1992) *Healthy Alliances* (London: King's Fund).

Powell, M. and Glendinning, C. (2002) 'Introduction'. In Glendinning, C., Powell, M. and Rummery, K. (eds) *Partnerships, New Labour and Governance* (Bristol: Policy Press), pp. 1–15.

Powell, M. and Moon, G. (2001) 'Health action zones: the Third Way of a new area-based policy', *Health and Social Care in the Community*, 9, 43–50.

Powles, J. and Gifford, J. (1993) 'Health of nations: lessons from Victoria, Australia', *BMJ*, 306, 125–7.

Prah Ruger, J. (2005) 'The changing role of the World Bank in global public health', *American Journal of Public Health*, 95(1), 65–70.

Prah Ruger, J. and Yach, D. (2005) 'Global functions at the World Health Organization', *BMJ*, 330, 1099–100.

Prime Minister's Strategy Unit (2004) *Alcohol Harm Reduction Strategy for England* (London: Cabinet Office).

Private Eye (2011) 'All aboard the GAVI train', *Private Eye*, 10–23 June, p. 28.

Public Health Alliance (1988) *Beyond Acheson* (Birmingham: Public Health Alliance).

Public Health Commission (2009) *We're All in it Together: Improving the Long Term Health of the Nation* (www.publichealthcommission.co.uk; accessed 21 November 2009).

Public Health for the NHS (2012) *Health and Social Care Bill Will Leave Public Health Compromised, Weaker and Less Safe*, press release, Thursday 5 March 2012.

Public Health Wales (2011) *National Workforce Development Plan for Public Health in Wales* (www. wales.nhs.uk/sitesplus/888/page/49008; accessed 29 May 2012).

Putnam, R. (1993) 'The prosperous community: social capital and public life' *American Prospect*, 13, 35–42.

Putnam, R. (2000) *Bowling Alone* (New York: Simon & Schuster).

Randall, E. (2001) *The European Union and Health Policy* (Basingstoke: Palgrave).

Raphael, D. (2008) 'Shaping public policy and population health in the United States: why is the public health community missing in action?', *International Journal of Health Services*, 38(1), 63–94.

Raphael, D. and Bryant T. (2006) 'The state's role in promoting population health: public health concerns in Canada, USA, UK and Sweden', *Health Policy*, 78, 39–55.

Rask, M., Worthington, R. and Lammi, M. (2011) *Citizen Participation in Global Environmental Governance* (London: Earthscan).

Reed, G. (2008) 'Cuba's primary health care revolution: 30 years on', *Bulletin of the World Health Organisation*, 86(5), 327–9.

Regional Voices (2012) *Influencing Local Commissioning for Health and Care: Guidance for the Voluntary and Community Sector* (Leeds: Regional Voices).

Reich, M. (2000) 'Public-private partnerships for public health', *Nature Medicine*, 6, 617–20.

Rhodes, R. (1997) *Understanding Governance: Policy Networks, Governance, Reflexivity, and Accountability* (Buckingham: Open University Press).

Richards, D. and Smith, M. (2002) *Governance and Public Policy in the UK* (Oxford: Oxford University Press).

Richmond Council for Voluntary Services (2011) *A Mapping for Richmond upon Thames* (Richmond: RCVS).

Ritchie, D., Parry, D., Gnich, W. and Platt, S. (2004) 'Issues of participation, ownership and empowerment in a community development programme: tackling smoking in a low income area of Scotland', *Health Promotion International*, 19(1), 51–9.

Rittel, H. and Webber, M. (1973) 'Dilemmas in a general theory of planning', *Policy Sciences*, 4, 155–69.

Roberts, J. (2008) *Partners or Instruments: Can the Compact Guard the Independence and Autonomy of Voluntary Organisations?* Voluntary Sector Working Paper No. 8 (London: London School of Economics and Political Science, Centre for Civil Society).

Robinson, O. (1994) *Ancient Rome: City Planning and Administration* (London: Taylor & Francis).

Rosen, G. (1993) *A History of Public Health* (ed. E. Fee) (New York: John Hopkins University Press).

Roussos, S. and Fawcett, S. (2000) 'A review of collaborative partnerships as a strategy for improving community health', *Annual Review of Public Health*, 21, 369–402.

Rowe, M. and Devanney, C. (2003) 'Partnership and the governance of regeneration', *Critical Social Policy*, 2(3), 375–97.

Rummery, K. (2002) 'Towards a theory of welfare partnerships'. In Glendinning, C., Powell, M. and Rummery, K. (eds) *Partnerships, New Labour and Governance* (Bristol: Policy Press).

Russell, H. (2005) *National Evaluation of Local Strategic Partnerships: Issues Paper. Voluntary and Community Sector Engagement in Local Strategic Partnerships* (London: ODPM).

Rydin, Y., Bleahu, A., Davies M., Davila, J., Friel, S. and De Grandis, G. (2012) 'Shaping cities for health: complexity in the planning of urban environments in the 21st century', *Lancet*, 379, 2079–108.

Salamon, L. and Anheier, H. (1997) *Defining the Non-profit Sector: A Cross-national Analysis* (Manchester: Manchester University Press).

Salay, R. and Lincoln, R. (2008) 'Health impact assessments in the European Union', *Lancet*, 372, 860–1.

Scottish Executive (2000) *Our National Health: A Plan for Action, a Plan for Change* (Edinburgh: Scottish Executive).

Scottish Executive (2003a) *Improving Health in Scotland: The Challenge* (Edinburgh: Scottish Executive).

Scottish Executive (2003b) *Partnership for Care: Scotland's Health White Paper* (Edinburgh: Scottish Executive).

Scottish Government (2007a) *Better Health, Better Care: A Discussion Document* (Edinburgh: Scottish Government).

Scottish Government (2007b) *Better Health, Better Care: Action Plan* (Edinburgh: Scottish Government).

Scottish Health Council (2013) 'Organisational change' (www.scottishhealthcouncil.org/about/organisational_change.aspx; accessed 30 May 2013).

Scottish Office (1991) *Health Education in Scotland: A National Policy Statement* (Edinburgh: HMSO).

Scottish Office (1992) *Scotland's Health: A Challenge To Us All* (Edinburgh: HMSO).

Scriven, A. (1998) *Alliances in Health Promotion: Theory and Practice* (Basingstoke: Palgrave).

Select Committee on Public Administration (2001) *Public Participation: Issues and Innovations. 6th Report 2000–1.* HC 373 (London: TSO).

Select Committee on Public Administration (2008a) *User Involvement in Public Services. 6th Report 2007–8.* HC 410 (London: TSO).

Select Committee on Public Administration (2008b) *Public Services and the Third Sector: Rhetoric and Reality. 11th Report Session 2007–08.* HC112. (London: TSO).

Select Committee on Public Administration (2011) *The Big Society. 17th Report Session 2010–12.* HC 902 (London: TSO).

Select Committee on Public Administration (2012) *The Big Society: Further Report with the Government Response to the Committee's Seventeenth Report of Session 2010–12. First Report 2012–13.* HC 98 (London: TSO).

Senate Committee on Social Affairs, Science and Technology (2003) *Reforming Health Protection and Promotion in Canada: Time to Act* (www.parl.gc.ca/Content/SEN/Committee/372/soci/rep/repfinnov03-e.htm; accessed 5 June 2013).

Sheard, S. and Donaldson, L. (2006) *The Nation's Doctor: The Role of the Chief Medical Officer 1855–1998* (Oxford: Radcliffe Medical Press).

Simon, P. and Fielding, J. (2006) 'Public health and business: a partnership that makes cents', *Health Affairs*, 25(4), 1029–39.

Single European Act (1987) *Official Journal of the European Communities*, 29 June 1987, L169.

Skelcher, C. (2000) 'Changing images of the state: overloaded, hollowed out, congested', *Public Policy and Administration*, 15(3), 3–19.

Skidmore, P., Bound, K. and Lownsbrough, L. (2006) *Community Participation: Who Benefits?* (York: Joseph Rowntree Foundation).

Sklair, L. and Miller, D. (2010) 'Capitalist globalisation, corporate social responsibility and social policy', *Critical Social Policy*, 30(2), 472–95.

Smith, A. and Jacobson, B. (1988) *The Nation's Health: A Strategy for the 1990s* (London: King's Fund).

Smith, K., Bambra, C., Joyce, K., Perkins, N., Hunter, D. and Blenkinsopp, E. (2009) 'Partners in health? A systematic review of the impact of organisational partnerships on public health outcomes in England between 1997 and 2008', *Journal of Public Health*, 31(2), 210–21.

Smith, R., Beaglehole, R., Woodward, D. and Drager, N. (2003) *Global Public Goods for Health: A Health Economic and Public Health Perspective* (Oxford: Oxford University Press).

Smith, R., Chanda, R. and Tangcharoensathien, V. (2009) 'Trade in health-related services', *Lancet*, 373, 593–601.

Snape, S. (2004) 'Partnerships between health and local government: the local government policy context'. In Snape, S. and Taylor, P. (eds) *Partnerships Between Health and Local Government* (London: Frank Cass), pp. 73–98.

South, J., Meah, A., Bagnall, A., Kinsella, K., Branney, P., White, J. et al. (2010) *People in Public Health: A Study of Approaches to Develop and Support People in Public Health Roles*. (Southampton: National Institute for Health Research).

South, J., White, J., and Gamsu, M. (2012) *People-Centred Public Health* (Bristol: Policy Press).

Spiegel, J. and Yassi, A. (2004) 'Lessons from the margins of globalization: appreciating the Cuban health paradox', *Journal of Public Health Policy*, 25, 85–110.

Spiegel, J., Alegret, M., Clair, V., Pagliccia, N., Martinez, B. and Bonet, M. (2012) 'Intersectoral action for health at a municipal level in Cuba', *International Journal of Public Health*, 57(1), 15-23.

Stahl, T., Wismar, M., Ollila, E., Lahtinen, E. and Leppo, K. (2006) *Health in All Policies: Prospects and Potentials* (Helsinki: Ministry of Social Affairs and Health).

Stoker, G. (1998) 'Governance as theory: five propositions', *International Social Science Journal*, 50(155), 17–28.

Stone, D. (2012) *The Growing Public Health Crisis and How to Address It* (Oxford: Radcliffe Medical Press).

Storey, M., Boyd, G. and Dowd, J. (1999) 'Voluntary agreements with industry'. In Carraror, C. and Leveque, F. (eds) *Voluntary Approaches in Environmental Policy* (Dordrecht: Kluwer Academic Publishers), pp. 187–207.

Strategic Review of Health Inequalities in England (2010) *Fair Society: Healthy Lives* (London: DH).

Stuckler, D. and Basu, S. (2009) 'The International Monetary Fund's effects on global health: before and after the 2008 financial crisis', *International Journal of Health Studies*, 39(4), 771–81.

Stuckler, D., Basu, S. and McKee, M. (2011) 'Commentary UN high level meeting on non-communicable diseases: an opportunity for whom?', *BMJ*, 343, d5336, 23 August (accessed 31 May 2012).

Sturchio, J. and Goel, A. (2012) *The Private-sector Role in Public Health* (Washington: Centre for Strategic and International Studies).

Sullivan, H. and Skelcher, C. (2002) *Working Across Boundaries: Collaboration in Public Services* (Basingstoke: Palgrave).

Sustain (2005) *Social Enterprise for Community Food Projects: A Policy Briefing Paper* (London: Sustain).

Tam, H. (1998) *Communitarianism: A New Agenda for Politics and Citizenship* (Basingstoke: Macmillan).

Taylor, B., Mathers, J., Atfield, T. and Parry, J. (2011) 'What are the challenges to the Big Society in maintaining lay involvement in health improvement and how can they be met?', *Journal of Public Health*, 33(1), 5–10.

Taylor, M. (2003) *Public Policy in the Community* (Basingstoke: Palgrave).

Taylor, M. (2006) 'Communities in partnership: developing a strategic voice', *Social Policy and Society*, 5(2), 269–79.

Taylor, P. (1984) *The Smoke Ring: Tobacco, Money and Multi-National Politics* (London: Bodley Head).

Taylor, P., Peckham, S. and Turton, P. (1998) *A Public Health Model of Primary Care: From Concept to Reality* (Birmingham: Public Health Alliance).

Tervonen-Goncalves, L. and Lehto, J. (2004) 'Transfer of health for all policy: what, how and in which direction? A two case study', *Health Research Policy and Systems*, 2, 8.

Thaler, R. and Sunstein, C. (2009) *Nudge* (London: Penguin).

Thom, B., Herring, R., Bayley, M., and Waller, S. (2013) 'Partnerships: survey respondents' perceptions of inter-professional collaboration to address alcohol-related harms in England', *Critical Public Health*, 23(1), 62–76.

Tilson, H. and Berkowitz, B. (2006) 'The public health enterprise: examining our twenty first century policy challenges', *Health Affairs*, 24(4), 900.

Timmins, N. (2012) *Never Again? The Story of the Health and Social Care Act 2012* (London: King's Fund/Institute for Government).

Treaty on European Union (1992) *Official Journal of the European Communities*, C244, 31 August (http://europa.eu.int/en/record/mt/top.html; accessed 19 March 2007).

Treaty of Rome (1957) (http://ec.europa.eu/economy_finance/emu_history/documents/treaties/rometreaty2.pdf; accessed 14 January 2011).

Tritter, J. and McCallum, A. (2006) 'The snakes and ladders of user involvement: moving beyond Arnstein', *Health Policy*, 7, 156–68.

Tunstill, J., Allnock, D., Meadows, P. and McLeod, A. (2002) *Early Experiences of Implementing Sure Start Sure Start* (London: University of London, National Evaluation Team).

UN (United Nations) (1993) *Agenda 21: Earth Summit – The United Nations Programme of Action from Rio* (Geneva: UN).

UN (2007) *The UN Global Compact* (www.unglobalcompact.org; accessed 4 April 2012).

UN General Assembly (2000) *United Nations Millennium Declaration: Resolution Adopted by the General Assembly*. 55th session, 18 September 2000, A/res/55/2.

UN General Assembly (2009a) *63rd Session Agenda Item 44 Global Health and Foreign Policy*. 63/33.

UN General Assembly (2009b) *Official Records of the General Assembly Sixty Fourth Session Supplement 3*. A64/3/Rev 1, Ch3, para III.

UN General Assembly (2010) *Resolution A/RES/64/265 on Prevention and Control of Non-communicable Diseases*.

UN General Assembly (2012a) *Resolution Adopted By the General Assembly 66th Session 11 September 2012. The Future We Want*. A/RES/66/288.

UN General Assembly (2012b) *Resolution Adopted By the General Assembly 66th Session 19 September, 2011. Political Declaration of the High-level Meeting of the General Assembly on the Prevention and Control of Non-communicable Diseases*. A/RES/66/2.

UN General Assembly (2012c) *Note by the Secretary-General Transmitting the Report of the Director-General of the World Health Organization on Options for Strengthening and Facilitating Multisectoral Action for the Prevention and Control of Non-communicable Diseases Through Effective Partnership*. UN General Assembly 67th Session, 17 September 2012, A/67/373.

UN General Assembly (2012d) *Global Health and Foreign Policy*, 67th Session 6, December, A/67/l36.

Unwin, J. and Westland, P. (2000) *Health Action Zones: The Engagement of the Voluntary Sector* (London: Baring Foundation).

USDHHS (US Department of Health and Human Services) (1980) *Promoting Health/Preventing Disease: Objectives for the Nation* (Washington, DC: Public Health Service).

USDHHS (1991) *Healthy People 2000* (Washington, DC: Public Health Service).

USDHHS (2010) *Healthy People 2020* (http://www.healthypeople.gov/2020/default.aspx; accessed 5 July 2013).

US Surgeon General (1979) *Healthy People: The Surgeon General's Report on Health Promotion and Disease Prevention* (Washington, DC: US Office of Surgeon General).

Veenstra, G., Luginaah, I., Wakefield, S., Birch, S., Eyles, J. and Elliott, S. (2005) 'Who you know, where you live: social capital, neighbourhood and health', *Social Science and Medicine*, 60, 2799–818.

Voluntary Action Westminster (2010) *Reducing Health Inequality in Westminster: The Role of the Voluntary and Community Sector* (London: Voluntary Action Westminster).

Voluntary Health Scotland (2005) *Community Health Partnerships: Involving the Voluntary Sector*. Advice Note (Edinburgh: VHS).

Voluntary Health Scotland (2007) *Further Advice Note on the Role of Voluntary Sector Members of CHPs* (Edinburgh: VHS).

Voluntary Health Scotland (2009a) *Improving CHP Engagement with the Third Sector: A Survey of CHP General Managers by VHS* (Edinburgh: VHS).

Voluntary Health Scotland (2009b) *The Role of the Third Sector in Health Improvement within CHPs: A Sector Perspective* (Edinburgh: VHS).

Voluntary Health Scotland (2011) *Engaging with Scotland's Health Agenda: A Survey of Local Intermediary Bodies* (Edinburgh: VHS).

Wait, S. and Nolte, E. (2006) 'Public involvement in policies in health: exploring their conceptual basis', *Health Economics, Policy and Law*, 1, 149–62.

Wallace-Brown, G. and Harman, S. (2011) 'Preface: risk, perceptions of risk and global health governance', *Political Studies*, 59(4), 773–8.

Wanless, D. (2003) *The Review of Health and Social Care in Wales* (Cardiff: Welsh Assembly).

Wanless, D. (2004) *Securing Good Health for the Whole Population* (London: HM Treasury).

Wanless, D. (2007) *Our Future Health Secured* (London: King's Fund).

Warwick, P. (2007) 'The rise and fall of the patient forum', *British Journal of Healthcare Management*, 13(7), 250–4.

Watt, E., Ibe, O. and McLelland, N. (2010) *Study of Community Health Partnerships* (Edinburgh: Scottish Government Social Research).

Webster, C. (1996) *Government and Health Care*, Vol. II: *The National Health Service 1958–79* (London: HMSO).

Weeks, J., Aggleton, P., McKevitt, C., Parkinson, K. and Taylor-Laybourn, A. (1996) 'Community and contracts: tensions and dilemmas in the voluntary sector response to HIV and AIDS', *Policy Studies*, 17(2), 107–23.

Weightwatchers (2011) *Written Evidence from Weightwatchers' Health Committee 2010–11* (London: TSO).

Weiss, E., Anderson, R. and Lasker, R. (2002) 'Making the most of collaboration: exploring the relationship between partnership synergy and partnership functioning', *Health Education an Behaviour*, 29, 683–98.

Welsh Assembly Government (2002) *Wellbeing in Wales* (Cardiff: WAG).

Welsh Assembly Government (2003a) *Wales: A Better Country* (Cardiff: WAG).

Welsh Assembly Government (2003b) *Signposts Two: Putting Patient and Public Involvement into Practice* (Cardiff: WAG).

Welsh Assembly Government (2005) *Designed for Life: Creating World Class Health and Social Care for Wales in the 21st Century* (Cardiff: WAG).

Welsh Assembly Government (2006) *Making the Connections – Delivering Beyond Boundaries. Transforming Public Services in Wales* (Cardiff: WAG).

Welsh Assembly Government (2007) *A Shared Responsibility* (Cardiff: WAG).

Welsh Assembly Government (2008) *The Third Dimension: A Strategic Action Plan for the Voluntary Sector Scheme* (Cardiff, WAG).

Welsh Assembly Government (2009) *Our Healthy Future* (Cardiff: WAG).

Welsh Government (2012) *Patients' Voice for Wales: Proposals Following the Review of Community Health Councils* (Cardiff: WAG).

Welsh Office (1998) *Strategic Framework: Better Health, Better Wales* (Cardiff: Welsh Office).

Welsh Office/NHS Directorate (1989) *Welsh Health Planning Forum: Strategic Intent and Direction for the NHS in Wales* (Cardiff: Welsh Office).

Which? (2012) *Responsibility Deal: One Year On* (London: Which?).

White, C. (2011) 'Commercial sector has much to offer in improving health, says England's Chief Medical Officer' *BMJ*, 343, d4216, 4 July (accessed 25 July 2011).

White, J., South, J., Woodall, J. and Kinsella, K. (2010) *Altogether Better: Thematic Evaluation Community Health Champions and Empowerment* (Leeds: Leeds Metropolitan University, Centre for Health Promotion Research).

Whitehead, M. (2007) 'The architecture of partnerships: urban communities in the shadow of hierarchy', *Policy Press*, 35(1), 3–23.

WHO (World Health Organization) (1946) *Constitution: Basic Documents* (Geneva: WHO).

WHO (1981) *Global Health Strategy for Health for All by the Year 2000* (Geneva: WHO).

WHO (1986) *First International Conference on Health Promotion. The Move Towards a New Public Health: Ottawa Charter for Health Promotion, Ottawa Nov 17–21* (Ottawa: WHO/Health and Welfare Canada/Canadian Association for Public Health).

WHO (1988) *Second International Conference on Health Promotion: Adelaide Recommendations* (Adelaide: WHO/Australian Department of Community Services and Health).

WHO (1991) *Third International Conference on Health Promotion: Sundsvall Statement on Supportive Environments for Health* (Sundsvall: WHO/UNEP/Nordic Council of Ministers).

WHO (1997) *Fourth International Conference on Health Promotion: The Jakarta Declaration* (Jakarta: WHO).

WHO (1998a) *Health for All for the 21st Century* (Geneva: WHO).

WHO (1998b) *World Health Assembly Resolution WHA 51.12: Health Promotion.* 51st World Health Assembly (Geneva: WHO).

WHO (1999) *Public–Private Partnerships for Health: Report by the Director General.* Executive Boards 105th Session. EB 105/8 (London: WHO).

WHO (2000a) *The Fifth Global Conference on Health Promotion. Health Promotion: Bridging the Equity Gap, 5–9 June Mexico City* (www.who.int/healthpromotion/conferences/previous/mexico/en/hpr_mexico_report_en.pdf; accessed 21 May 2010).

WHO (2000b) *Guidelines on Working with the Private Sector To Achieve Health Outcomes. Report by the Secretariat.* EB 107/20 (Geneva: WHO).

WHO (2001) *Strategic Alliances: The Role of Civil Society in Health* (Geneva: WHO).

WHO (2002) *Global Strategy for Food Safety* (Geneva: WHO).

WHO (2003) *WHO Framework Convention on Tobacco Control* (Geneva: WHO).

WHO (2004) *Fifty-Seventh World Health Assembly, Provisional Agenda Item 12.6: Global Strategy on Diet, Physical Activity and Health* (Geneva: WHO).

WHO (2005) *The Bangkok Charter for Health Promotion in a Globalised World. 6th Global Conference on Health Promotion, Bangkok, Thailand 7–11 August* (www.who.int/healthpromotion/conferences/6gchp/hpr_050829_%20BCHP.pdf; accessed 21 May 2010).

WHO (2008a) *Prevention and Control of Non-Communicable Diseases: Implementation of the Global Strategy* (Geneva: WHO).

WHO (2008b) *2008–13 Action Plan for the Global Strategy for the Prevention and Control of Non-communicable Diseases* (Geneva: WHO).

WHO (2009) *Promoting Health and Development: Closing the Implementation Gap 7th Global Conference on Health Promotion. 26–30 October, Nairobi, Kenya* (Geneva: WHO).

WHO (2010a) *Partnerships.* World Health Assembly Resolution WHA 63.10, May (Geneva: WHO).

WHO (2010b) *Draft Global Strategy to Reduce the Harmful Use of Alcohol (revised version)* (Geneva: WHO).

WHO (2012a) *Effective Approaches for Strengthening Multisectoral Action for NCDs.* WHO Discussion Paper No. 1 (Geneva: WHO).

WHO (2012b) *Global Action Plan for the Prevention and Control of Non-communicable Diseases 2012–20. Zero Draft* (Geneva: WHO).

WHO/Government of South Australia (2010) *Adelaide Statement on Health in all Policies* (Geneva: WHO).

WHO/UNEP (2011) 'Health and Environment Links Initiative' (www.who.int/heli/en/index.html; accessed 11 January 2011).

WHO/UNICEF (1978) *Declaration of Alma Ata. Report of the International Conference on Primary Health Care* (Geneva: WHO/UNICEF).

WHO Commission on Macroeconomics and Health (2001) *Macroeconomics and Health: Investing in Health for Economic Development* (chair J. Sachs) (Geneva: WHO).

WHO Commission on Social Determinants of Health (2008) *Closing the Gap in a Generation: Health Equity Through Action on the Social Determinants of Health* (Geneva: WHO).

WHO Regional Office for Europe (1985) *Targets for Health for All: Targets in Support of the European Regional Strategy for Health for All* (Copenhagen: WHO).

WHO Regional Office for Europe (1988) *Healthy Nutrition: Preventing Nutrition-Related Disease in Europe* (Copenhagen: WHO).

WHO Regional Office for Europe (1990) *Health and Environment: Charter and Commentary* (Copenhagen: WHO Europe).

WHO Regional Office for Europe (1993a) *European Alcohol Action Plan* (Copenhagen: WHO).

WHO Regional Office for Europe (1993b) *Action Plan for a Tobacco Free Europe* (Copenhagen: WHO Regional Office for Europe).

WHO Regional Office for Europe (1993c) *Health for All Targets: The Health Policy for Europe* (Copenhagen: WHO).

WHO Regional Office for Europe (1999a) *Health 21: The Health for All Policy Framework for the Twenty First Century* (Copenhagen: WHO Europe).

WHO Regional Office for Europe (1999b) *Charter on Transport, Environment and Health* (Copenhagen: WHO Europe).

WHO Regional Office for Europe (2000a) *First Action Plan for Food and Nutrition Policy* (Copenhagen: WHO).

WHO Regional Office for Europe (2000b) *European Alcohol Action Plan 2000–2005* (Copenhagen: WHO Europe).

WHO Regional Office for Europe (2001) *Declaration on Young People and Alcohol.* Adopted in Stockholm on 21 February 2001 (Copenhagen: WHO Europe).

WHO Regional Office for Europe (2002) *Review of National Finnish Health Promotion Policies and Recommendations for the Future.* (Copenhagen: WHO Europe).

WHO Regional Office for Europe (2004) *Children's Environment and Health Action Plan for Europe. Fourth Ministerial Conference on Environment and Health* (Copenhagen: WHO Europe).

WHO Regional Office for Europe (2006a) *European Charter on Counteracting Obesity. WHO European Ministerial Conference on Counteracting Obesity, Diet and Physical Activity for Health, Istanbul, Turkey, 15–17 November* (Copenhagen: WHO Europe).

WHO Regional Office for Europe (2006b) *Framework for Alcohol Policy in the WHO European Region* (Copenhagen: WHO Regional Office for Europe).

WHO Regional Office for Europe (2010) *Parma Declaration on Environment and Health. Fifth Ministerial Conference on Environment and Health. Parma, Italy, 1–12 March* (Copenhagen: WHO Regional Office for Europe).

WHO Regional Office for Europe (2011) *Action Plan for the Implementation of the European Strategy for the Prevention and Control of Non-communicable Diseases 2012–16* (Copenhagen: WHO Regional Office for Europe).

WHO Regional Office for Europe (2012a) *Addressing the Social Determinants of Health: The Urban Dimension and the Role of Local Government* (Copenhagen: WHO Regional Office for Europe).

WHO Regional Office for Europe (2012b) *Health 2020: A European Policy Framework Supporting Action Across Government and Society for Health and Well-being* (Copenhagen: WHO Regional Office for Europe).

Wicklander, M. (2006) 'Implementing and evaluating the National Healthy School Program in England', *Journal of School Nursing*, 22(5), 250–8.

Widdus, R. (2001) 'Public-private partnerships for health: their main targets, their diversity and their future directions', *Bulletin of the World Health Organisation*, 79, 713–20.

Wildridge, V., Childs, S., Cawthra, L. and Madge, B. (2004) 'How to create successful partnerships: a review of the literature', *Health Information and Libraries Journal*, 21(S1), 3–19.

Wilkes, J. (2010) *A National Skills Framework for the Voluntary Sector* (Sheffield: Skills Third Sector).

Wilkinson, D. and Appleby, E. (1999) *Holistic Government: Implementing Joined Up Action on the Ground* (Bristol: Policy Press).

Williams, N. (1999) 'Modernising government: policy making within Whitehall', *Political Quarterly*, 70, 452–9.

Williams, P. (2011) 'The life and times of the Boundary Spanner', *Journal of Integrated Care*, 19(3), 26–33.

Williamson, C. (1992) *Whose Standards? Consumer and Professional Standards in Health Care* (Buckingham: Open University Press).

Willmott, M. (2012) *A Case Study of Voluntary Organisations' Participation in Local Health Policy in England*. Thesis submitted for the degree of Doctor of Philosophy, April 2012, London School of Hygiene and Tropical Medicine.

Wills, J. and Ellison, G. (2007) 'Integrating services for public health: challenges facing multidisciplinary working', *Public Health*, 121, 546–8.

Wismar, M., Blau, J., Ernst, K. and Figueras, J. (2007) *The Effectiveness of Health Impact Assessment: Scope and Limitations of Supporting Decision Making in Europe* (Copenhagen: WHO/European Observatory on Health Systems and Policies).

Wistow, G. (2012) 'Still a fine mess? Local government and the NHS 1962 to 2012', *Journal of Integrated Care*, 20(2), 101–14.

Wohl, A.S. (1984) *Endangered Lives, Public Health in Victorian Britain* (London: Unwin Methuen).

Wood, B. (2000) *Patient Power?* (Buckingham: Open University Press).

Woodall, J, Raine, G., South, G. and Warwick-Booth, L. (2010) *Empowerment, Health and Wellbeing: Evidence Review* (Leeds: Centre for Health Promotion Research).

World Bank (2011) *The Growing Danger of Non-communicable Disease* (World Bank).

WTO (1994) *The WTO Agreement on the Application of Sanitary and Phytosanitary Measures* (Geneva: WTO).

Wyatt, M. (2002) 'Partnership in health and social care: the implications of government guidance in the 1990s in England, with particular reference to voluntary organisations', *Policy and Politics*, 30(2), 167–82.

Yach, D. and Bettcher, D. (1998a) 'The globalisation of public health. Part I. Threats and opportunities', *American Journal of Public Health*, 8(5), 735–8.

Yach, D. and Bettcher, D. (1998b) 'The globalisation of public health. Part II. The convergence of self-interest and altruism', *American Journal of Public Health*, 8(5), 738–41.

Yamey, G. (2002a) 'Why does the world still need WHO?', *BMJ*, 325, 1294–8.

Yamey, G. (2002b) 'WHO's management: struggling to reform a "fossilised bureaucracy"', *BMJ*, 325, 1170–3.

Ziglio, E., Hagard, S. and Brown, C. (2005) 'Health promotion development in Europe: barriers and new opportunities'. In Scriven, E. and Garman, S. (eds) *Promoting Health: Global Perspectives* (Basingstoke: Palgrave), pp. 229–38.

Zimmeck, M., Rochester, C. and Rushbrooke, B. (2011) *Use It or Lose It: A Summative Evaluation of the Compact* (London: Commission for the Compact).

Index